The Handbook of Consultation Psychiatry:
A Roadmap to Psychiatry in the General Hospital

By James L. Stinnett, MD
Emeritus Professor of Psychiatry
Perelman School of Medicine
University of Pennsylvania

DEDICATION

This volume is dedicated to my wife, Carol,
in gratitude for the wonderful life we share.

Acknowledgements

This Handbook could not have been produced without the help of the people mentioned below:

The most important contributors to this volume are the many faculty colleagues, residents, Fellows, and students who have worked with me over the past 25 years on the Psychiatry Consultation Service at the Hospital of the University of Pennsylvania. One of the many valuable benefits of the privilege of practicing Medicine in an academic medical center is the opportunity to discuss ideas with trainees and faculty colleagues in an atmosphere of rigorous intellectual discipline that promotes and encourages a free exchange of ideas and a critical appraisal of those ideas. It is this atmosphere that has provided me with the opportunity to discuss and refine many of the ideas in this volume before committing them to paper. If any of my former trainees or faculty colleagues were to read this Handbook, I am certain they will recognize some of their ideas that have been woven into the fabric of this work. I am greatly indebted to all of them, and I wish it were possible to individually acknowledge their specific contributions.

I wish to thank Dr. Dwight Evans whose tenure as Chair of the Dept. of Psychiatry of the University of Pennsylvania School of Medicine spanned the period of time beginning with the first edition of this volume throughout the intervening years to the present. Dr. Evans granted me a sabbatical leave 10 years ago which provided me the opportunity to write the first volume of this Handbook.

I wish to thank Dr. Henry Bleier who has been a valued colleague, a fellow consultation psychiatrist, and, most important, my very good friend. Much of the material in this Handbook is a distillate of countless discussions he and I have had over lunch and in the classroom. His keen intellect, infectious energy and curiosity, and his encouragement have had an enormous impact on how I think about many of the topics discussed in this volume.

I also wish to acknowledge Dr. Robert Weinrieb who was my successor after my retirement, now Chief of the Psychiatry Consultation Service at the Hospital of the University of Pennsylvania. He ably continued and improved the teaching qualities of the service for generations of medical students, residents, and Fellows who, each year, rotate through this service as part of their educational experience.

TABLE OF CONTENTS

Introduction

This is a "handbook," meant to be both easily accessible and practical. It's intended to convey information to assist the practitioner in "how to do" psychiatric consultations on medical/surgical patients in both hospital and ambulatory clinical settings. This handbook is intended for residents in Psychiatry who are learning how to do psychiatric consultations on patients who are medically ill and hospitalized in medical and surgical settings. In addition, it is my hope that Fellows in Psychosomatic Medicine/Consultation Psychiatry and medical students doing their clerkships on psychiatry consultation services will also find it helpful.

This volume is not meant to be a textbook, nor does it have any pretensions of being so. Unlike a textbook, it will not provide a summary of the relevant knowledge related to a specific topic, but will instead discuss how to understand a particular clinical issue and how to use that understanding to develop an effective clinical intervention to help the patient and the clinical team caring for the patient. The knowledge base that supports those conceptualizations and interventions will be selectively summarized and, in a limited fashion, referenced.

Chapter 1: Overview

Consultation Psychiatry is a recognized subspecialty of Psychiatry which is operationally defined by three characteristics:

A. A Process
The *process* of providing a consultation to a colleague regarding a patient.

B. Geography
The consultation process takes place in a medical/surgical setting (in a general medical-surgical hospital or ambulatory setting) and not in a psychiatric setting.

C. Patients
The patient population evaluated by consultation psychiatrists (CP) have medical and/or surgical illness. They may also have co-morbid psychiatric disorders that are related, or unrelated, to their primary medical condition.

A. The Consultation Process

The process of providing a psychiatric consultation is shaped by two parameters: the medical/surgical clinical setting and the time available to perform the consultation. Most patients admitted to general hospitals have a high degree of clinical acuity and are very sick. The pace of disease and the diagnostic and clinical interventions required usually progress at a more rapid rate than in the usual psychiatric settings. In addition, there are limitations on the amount of time the consultant has available to spend with an individual patient.

The limitation on time is a function of two factors: one, that due to acute physical illness, patients often do not feel well enough to sustain the amount of attention required to participate in a lengthy psychiatric interview and, two, the very high prevalence of psychiatric morbidity in hospitalized medical-surgical patients which results in a high number of requests for psychiatric consultation. This falls on a limited number of psychiatric consultants available to provide this service, so the issue of time is paramount. Most psychiatry consultation services are understaffed relative to the demand for their services, so for the reasons mentioned above, there is rarely enough time to do a thorough and detailed evaluation of each patient.

The twin realities of high acuity/high volume and limited time exert a powerful Darwinian pressure on the consultation psychiatrist to develop a clinical process that is tightly targeted at those psychiatric issues that are most important in the overall clinical context of the patient's medical/surgical problem and those treatment interventions that can be provided in the limited time available. This issue has led some experienced consultation psychiatrist to characterize the clinical work they do as "battlefield psychiatry."

B. Geography:

The consultation psychiatrist practices on someone else's "clinical turf"; in this case, in a medical-surgical hospital or ambulatory care setting. There are a number of interesting metaphors that have been used to describe this situation and I think the most accurate one is to see the consultation psychiatrist as an ambassador who represents his country (Psychiatry) in a foreign land (in-patient hospital or ambulatory medical-surgical setting). Like any effective "ambassador," the consultation psychiatrist must understand and be at home in the culture of the country he is posted to. He must understand and be able to speak the "language" of the country to which he is assigned. And most of all, he must have the "respect" (as a physician) of those with whom he interacts.

Regardless of the metaphor, it's important to emphasize that as a consultation psychiatrist you are functioning in a different clinical setting (medical-surgical) and helping someone else's patient. This is what gives Consultation Psychiatry its unique status.

C. Specific Disorders:

The consultation psychiatrist evaluates a group of psychiatric disorders and clinical issues that are seen with greater frequency in, and in some cases are unique to, medical-surgical clinical settings than in psychiatric settings, e.g. Delirium, Somatic Symptom Disorders, Factitious Physical Disorders, and Mood Disorders that exist in the clinical context of severe physical illness.

These three characteristics, the consultation process, the geography, and the patient population, are what give the discipline of Consultation Psychiatry its unique characteristics.

There are many benefits to doing consultation psychiatry. As mentioned above, you encounter a group of very interesting disorders and clinical issues that are largely context specific and seldom seen in more traditional psychiatric settings. Skills learned doing psychiatric consultations where there is an imperative to doing clinical examinations that are tightly targeted in a short period of time can be generalized to other psychiatric settings, such as emergency rooms. In addition, as more non-medically trained mental health professionals enter the field of mental health, consultation psychiatrists will always be able to claim the unique status of the medically trained mental health professional.

In the past decade, Psychosomatic Medicine-Consultation Psychiatry has gained recognition by the American Psychiatric Association and the American Board of Medical Specialties as a fully recognized subspecialty of Psychiatry. As such, it has its own subspecialty journals like *Psychosomatics* and *General Hospital Psychiatry*, its own professional organization, the Academy of Psychosomatic Medicine, and its own Fellowship training programs with subspecialty certification exams.

Chapter 2: Educational Objectives

1) The <u>skill</u> of providing an efficient and effective psychiatric consultation
2) The acquisition of a solid <u>knowledge</u> base of the types of psychiatric disorders seen in a general medical-surgical hospital
3) The development of appropriate <u>attitudes</u> and <u>behaviors</u> that are necessary to function effectively as a consultation psychiatrist when interacting with our physician colleagues.

The appropriate <u>skill</u> involves learning how to provide a <u>brief, focused</u> psychiatric assessment (not a comprehensive assessment), and how to communicate the results of that assessment in a concise verbal communication to the staff caring for the patient and in a written consultation on the patient's chart.

This skill can be conceptualized as the Brief Focused Psychiatric Assessment (BFPA) and should take only 20-30 minutes to conduct. It is important to emphasize that this is a <u>screening</u> assessment, not a comprehensive, diagnostic psychiatric interview. There are two primary reasons for this type of interview: one, most hospitalized patients are far too ill to be questioned in depth about details of their past or present psychiatric history and, two, most, if not all, psychiatric consultants working in a general medical-surgical in-patient setting work under extreme time pressures with a high demand for their clinical services and little time available to meet that demand.

The primary objective of this type of assessment is to identify the current psychiatric issues likely to affect the morbidity and mortality of the patient's current medical issues which are the main reason for their being in the hospital in the first place. Of secondary importance is "case finding" or the detection of psychiatric problems that may affect the patient's well-being and function independent of their current medical problems. This can usually be postponed to a time when the patient is not seriously ill with a medical or surgical illness, so the consultation psychiatrist can be thought of as functioning in a "triage" mode, i.e., addressing those issues that are most critical at the time and those issues that are most likely to have an impact on the patient's current medical state.

The BFPA is composed of two parts: 1) history and 2) a mental status examination. The primary focus of the history is on <u>current</u> symptoms. This has to do with the issue of priorities. Your primary, but not exclusive, concern is to address the psychiatric symptoms and signs that are most relevant to the patient's current medical/surgical problem, those that are the basis for the hospitalization. This overarching objective shapes the history and the type of mental status examination that you perform. The other factor that influences the type of history you take is the enormous time pressure that characterizes the process of consultation psychiatry. This explains the emphasis on elucidating what's happening <u>now</u> rather than what's happened in the <u>past</u>. There are some important exceptions to this emphasis on the current at the expense of the past, including recent history of substance use and suicide attempts. The focus of the history can often be guided by the initial consultation request and allows the interviewer to "laser in" on the issues underlying the questions asked by the patient's primary care team. The questions asked don't always turn out to be the most important, but it does help you to get started.

Use the A-B-C mnemonic to guide the gathering of historical data.

"A" is for the psychological domain of **<u>affect/emotion</u>**. The three main emotions and affects of importance in this clinical setting are <u>fear</u> (anxiety), <u>anger</u>, and <u>sadness</u> (depression). These three emotional states obviously do not encompass the entire spectrum of human emotional experience, but they are the ones most often associated with physical illness, and they are the ones that may add to the morbidity of the patient's current medical illness.

"B" is for <u>Behavior</u>. The issue here is not to take a comprehensive inventory of all clinically significant behaviors but to focus on those that are most likely to affect the outcome of the patient's current illness. Some examples of behaviors relevant to this clinical context are:

1) Treatment non-compliance.
2) Substance use (intoxication or withdrawal).
3) Angry, threatening, or disruptive behavior that interferes with care.
4) Suicidal or self-harm behaviors.

"C" is for <u>cognition</u>. It's important to know if the patient is experiencing any subjective, troubling cognitive symptoms such as feeling confused, paranoid, or experiencing hallucinations.

It's important to know how much history to take and how much NOT to take. This skill is acquired by experience and difficult to teach. Some past psychiatric history is important to know because it will probably affect the patient's current state. Perhaps the most significant example of this is the patient's substance use or recent or current use of CNS active medications.

It is also important to always be aware of the guiding principle of a psychiatric consultation history, that your clinical task is NOT to perform a <u>comprehensive</u> psychiatric <u>diagnostic</u> evaluation, but to laser in on the immediate problems, symptoms, and signs are that are most likely to affect the patient's current state while in the hospital.

Mental Status Examination

This part of the BFPA is also shaped by the factors outlined above. The emphasis is on <u>brief</u> and <u>focused</u>. Time and patient stamina will not permit a detailed and exhaustive mental status exam. As with the history, the mental status exam can also be framed in the **"A-B-C" format.**

AFFECT

The important parameters of affect are:

1) <u>Content</u> -- Anger, Fear/Anxiety, Apathy, and Sadness.
2) <u>Range</u> -- Full, Constricted, or Flat
3) <u>Volume</u>
4) <u>Appropriateness</u> to thought content and the current clinical situation.

5) <u>Modulation</u> --This is an important part of the mental status exam because it is this aspect that is very sensitive to a range of neuro-psychiatric disorders that may be seen in various physical illnesses. Modulation refers to the complex process by which the brain modulates or calibrates the expression of affect. This process is often thought to be analogous to a "dimmer" switch used to control the amount of light in a room. A defect in the brain's ability to modulate affect may be expressed as "labile" affect or as described by the colorful and very expressive phrase "affective Incontinence," which refers to the person who, at the slightest mention of something sad, will quickly burst into tears or at the slightest frustration becomes enraged.

BEHAVIOR

The behaviors that are of primary importance in the mental status exam of the hospitalized, physically ill patient are those that have a high probability of compromising the medical and surgical care of the physically ill patient. With the pressure of time, one seldom has the luxury of observing all the possible behaviors that might be diagnostically relevant, so it's important to focus on those that are most relevant to the clinical context of a seriously ill patient.

With that caveat in mind, it's important to note the presence or absence of certain <u>motor behaviors</u> such as agitation or non-purposeful, stereotyped behaviors that might compromise care, e.g. the agitated ICU patient who has tubes, lines, and monitors that must be protected from accidental or intentional disruption. It may be important for certain post surgical patients to remain very still to protect the surgical site. Certain

Interpersonal behaviors have the potential to interfere seriously in the care of the patient. Examples are the hostile and aggressive patient whose behavior has the potential of alienating the medical and nursing staff on whom they are so dependent for their care. Non-compliance behaviors with both diagnostic and therapeutic procedures are of obvious clinical importance.

COGNITION

There are many neuro-cognitive functions that one can assess when performing a mental status exam; however, the functions that are of most significance to the hospitalized patient with a medical-surgical illness are:

1. Level of Consciousness.

Coma. No response to stimulation (sensory input).
Stupor. No response to "ambient" sensory stimuli, but a variable degree of responsiveness with active, vigorous sensory stimulation.
Lethargy. The normal state of sleep deprivation (as seen in many residents).
Normal
Hyper-Alert. A disproportionate, high amplitude verbal or motor response to minimal or ambient sensory stimulation.

2. Attention.

This neuro-cognitive function is difficult to operationally describe. It has three components:

Selection of relevant sensory input from the "field" of sensory input.
Locking onto the sensory input that has been selected and maintaining that "locked on" state in the face of competing ambient sensory stimulation.
Unlocking and attaching to another more context-relevant sensory stimulus when appropriate. Like level of consciousness, attention is very sensitive to subtle impairments of brain function.

3. Memory. Both short and long-term memory should be assessed.

4. Orientation. This refers to the complex neuro-cognitive process of orienting the self to external, objective reality. The usual dimensions of orientation that are tested are time, place, and person. In a hospitalized, acutely ill patient some of these dimensions may not be relevant. For instance, in today's medical culture with many different doctors and nurses caring for the ill patient, it may be very difficult for even the well-oriented patient to be oriented to a "person," i.e., their doctor. In a hospital, each day has its own monotonous rhythm with little that differentiates it from other days, so it may be understandably difficult for a patient to know if it's a Wednesday or Friday or the 3rd dor the 5th of the month. It is more clinically useful to know if the patient is oriented to "purpose," i.e., why they are in the hospital, or what is wrong with them, and whether they have intact circadian orientation, i.e., do they know if it is morning, afternoon, or night time.

5. Perception. Determine if there are abnormalities of perception, specifically hallucinations. In addition to the usual questions about visual and auditory hallucinations, inquire about the presence of olfactory, gustatory, tactile, and proprioceptive hallucinations since these are occasionally encountered in patients who have various types of physical brain pathology, e.g., substance withdrawal states or ictal and post-ictal phenomena.

6. Thought Process and Content. These cognitive functions are assessed in the usual way to determine if psychotic thinking is present.

7. Insight/Judgement/Appreciation of Illness. This is important to determine, particularly if there is a question about the cognitive capacity to make medical decisions. This aspect of the mental status exam will be discussed in much greater detail later in the chapter on Decision Making Capacity.

The primary educational objective of a rotation on a psychiatry consultation service is the development of certain skill sets, of which the **Brief Focused Psychiatric Assessment (BFPA)** described above is the most important. There are additional skills and attitudes that must be mastered and they parallel the unfolding of the consultation process over time, as described below.

1. <u>The Consultation Request.</u>
The consultation process begins with receiving the request for a consultation from a colleague. Your colleague is working under the same intense time pressures as you are, and you need to be as respectful of their time as you want them to be of yours, so try to quickly and succinctly clarify the question your colleague wants addressed and resist the impulse to ask your colleague a number of questions regarding the psychiatric history and mental status of the patient. That is your job.

It is, however, helpful to ask a few pertinent questions regarding the medical/surgical condition of the patient. There are times when the request for one more consultation during a very busy day for an overworked resident or attending may seem unwarranted and overwhelming, which occasionally gives rise to the "bogus consult" complaint on the part of the consultant psychiatrist. This complaint usually arises from the assumption that the question being asked can be handled just as well by the physician asking for the consult without involving an equally overworked consultant. Regardless of the possible legitimacy of this conclusion, it is important to put yourself in the shoes of the colleague who is requesting your help. Your colleague may not realize or fully appreciate that you think they can answer this question satisfactorily, and they may want a bit of "hand holding" by a specialist to make sure they are doing the right thing by the patient, so don't waste time complaining about a possible "bogus consultation." Just help your colleague and do the consultation.

When complaining about the "bogus" consultation request, remind yourself of the many times you have asked for a medical consult on one of your psychiatric in-patients. The medical consultant may feel that you should be able to answer this question yourself. After all, didn't you go to medical school? Can't you diagnose Hypertension? Don't you remember how to start anti-hypertension treatment? Of course you can, but you may just want a little hand-holding just to be sure you're doing the right thing by your patient.

Before ending the communication requesting the consultation, be sure to ask the physician requesting the consultation if s/he has notified the patient of the consultation request and has obtained the patient's agreement. This is not only a matter of common courtesy, but the patient's acquiescence to the consultation is necessary, particularly if they will receive a bill for any portion of the fee not covered by insurance.

2. Review of the Chart

Before seeing the patient, review the patient's chart. This may be a daunting process, particularly if the patient has been hospitalized for a long time and has a lengthy chart. Keeping in mind the always present time constraints, it may suffice to review the admission note and skip to the most recent progress notes in order to get the gist of the current clinical issues. Of utmost importance is to review the most recent labs, brain imaging, and current medications with particular focus on those medications that may have CNS effects.

3. Evaluation of the Patient

Introduce yourself to the patient and identify yourself as a psychiatrist who has been asked by the patient's physician to evaluate them. Ask the patient if they have been informed that a psychiatric consultation has been requested by their physician and if they are agreeable to participate in the evaluation. If they have not been informed that a psychiatrist was asked to perform a consultation, I prefer to briefly explain the reason for the consultation and to explain very succinctly what you will be doing, e.g. asking a few questions about how they are thinking and feeling about their current illness. Many patients who have never seen a psychiatrist or who may be psychologically unsophisticated may have unrealistic ideas of what a psychiatrist does.

They may think you are going to ask a lot of very personal questions about their childhood or their dreams or their sex lives, and these thoughts may be very threatening to them. If you couch your questions in the context of their current physical illness, it may not appear threatening, and they may be willing to cooperate with you even if they have not been informed of your visit beforehand.

After you have done the BFPA, discuss what you plan to do with the information you've obtained. I tell the patient that I am going to write a brief note, with very few details, in their hospital chart and have a conversation with their physician(s) regarding my clinical impressions and recommendations for treatment. I make it clear that the treatment team will make the final determination as to whether to implement my recommendations and I tell the patient that I will recommend that their doctor discuss those recommendations with them. I mention that I will try -- and don't promise this unless you are sure you will be able to do it -- to make a follow up visit to see how they are responding to any treatment I might recommend. Before leaving, ask the patient if they have any questions about your visit with them.

The above recommendations presuppose that the patient's mental status is clear and functioning well enough to understand what I am discussing with them. In certain situations, when this is not the case, e.g., psychosis, delirium, or coma, what you discuss with the patient must be tempered by what you think the patient can comprehend.

4. Written Consultation.
After your consultation with the patient is finished, communicate your findings and recommendations to the referring physician. It is most efficient to do this first by phone, describing your impression of what your clinical impression is and what your recommendations are. There is a widespread tendency to "over talk" this aspect of the communication. You are busy and your colleague is busy, and neither of you has the time to waste talking about and listening to information that may not be relevant to the two most pressing questions --what is wrong, and what to do about it.
After speaking with the referring physician, write a brief note in the patient's hospital record. There is a tendency to "over-write" the consult, and busy house officers and attendings do not have the time nor the interest in reading details of the history and MSE. They just want to know what's wrong and what to do about it. I recommend inverting the

usual narrative flow that all physicians have been taught, i.e., describing the history, then the exam, labs, results of diagnostic tests, followed by the diagnostic impression and treatment. Instead, start the written note with the Impression, followed by the treatment recommendations, and then a brief description of the relevant history and objective data (MSE, labs, meds, diagnostic tests). This way the busy reader of your note can get the crucial information (impression and treatment) first, like a "headline." If they're interested, they can read further.

This approach can be remembered by the acronym, **"IPSO": Impression, Plan, Subjective data (history), and Objective data.** Also, try to develop the habit of NOT summarizing in the written consult a lot of clinical data that the referring physician already knows. This is just a waste of time.

Many hospitals or providers will have a preprinted (either paper or EMR) format for the written consultation note. There are two "drivers" of this type of format. One is to prompt the consultant to fill in certain clinical data domains. The other is to use that data to support a certain level of clinical activity to justify a billing code level. The problem with these prompts is that it pushes the consultant to acquire and convey clinical data that may not be necessary to guide treatment for the immediate clinical issue. The effort to encourage and support a higher level of intervention, thereby justifying a higher billing code, raises an important ethical issue. Doing this, when it's not absolutely necessary to affect treatment outcome, is not <u>fraudulent</u>, because you've actually done what you've documented; but it is <u>wasteful</u>. You have wasted your time, the patient's time and energy, and money (insurance or the patient's) by doing work that does not add value to the clinical outcome. Wastefulness is a major and widespread problem in our healthcare system, and each of us has the responsibility to manage scarce health care resources by eliminating waste.

5. Follow Up.
The follow up of patients on a busy consultation service is a complex balancing act driven by the scarcity of time. Ideally, all patients seen in consultation and for whom some type of treatment intervention

is started should have a follow up to determine if the treatment is working and, in the case of starting medications, to see if the patient is experiencing any troubling side effects. Once again, there is seldom enough time to see every patient in follow up. Certain groups of patients must be seen every day or even more than once a day, and these patients' psychiatric problems are so acute and severe that they pose a high risk of impacting the morbidity and mortality of the patient. Three examples of this group are patients who are suicidal, psychotic, or delirious.

Another extremely important aspect is arranging psychiatric follow up for patients after they are discharged. Any patient started on a psychopharmacologic agent while in the hospital must have psychiatric follow up to see whether the medication is effective. This is particularly an issue in today's hospital culture where patients are discharged very rapidly. Most consultation psychiatrists would not argue with this imperative, but they would say that it is not their job (a very time-consuming job which is not reimbursable). Most would state that arranging out-patient psychiatric follow up is the responsibility of the unit social worker or the responsibility of the patient's physician to arrange outpatient psychiatric follow up. The problem with this argument (no matter how valid) is that these staff are as hard pressed for time as you are and their knowledge of the complexities of access to mental health services is often woefully lacking.

Many patients are discharged on psychiatric medication without adequate outpatient follow up and often stay on psychotropic medications far past the point when they are no longer needed, thereby increasing the risk of side effects with no appreciable benefit. Or, they may prematurely stop their medication once it has run out and run the risk of a symptomatic relapse.
The psychiatry consultant must take some responsibility in making sure psychiatric follow up gets arranged, either by doing it himself, or by making sure somebody does it before the patient is discharged. After all, a cardiac patient who is started on a cardiac medication by a cardiology consultant while in the hospital would not be discharged without a follow up appointment with a cardiologist to monitor the response to the medication. A patient with a new onset seizure who

has been started on anticonvulsants would not be discharged from the hospital without outpatient follow up with a neurologist. Similarly, we should not discharge a psychiatric patient who has been started on a psychopharmacologic agent without making sure the patient has a follow up appointment with a psychiatrist.

As mentioned at the beginning of this chapter, there are three overarching educational objectives to master when doing psychiatric consultations in the general hospital: **skills, knowledge, and attitudes**. Up to this point, we have been discussing the specific **skills** that need to be mastered. In subsequent chapters, we will cover the **knowledge** content relative to the types of psychiatric problems and disorders that are often seen on a psychiatry consultation service. We will now move to a discussion of the appropriate **attitudes** to develop to become a competent consultation psychiatrist.

Attitudes

There is a set of attitudes and "clinical reflexes" that vary in important ways from those developed in different clinical settings, e.g., in-patient psychiatric units and psychiatric outpatient settings. This difference is determined by the unique nature of functioning as a consultant and not as the patient's primary physician. In this capacity, you have two obligations: 1. the welfare of the patient, and, 2. to assist the colleague who has requested the consultation. The primary attitude and behavior, on the part of the consulting psychiatrist, that must be shaped is that of availability and helpfulness.

This brings to mind the famous statement, attributed to Sir William Osler, concerning the three paramount attributes of an excellent physician --"availability, affability, and ability...in that order." It is important to be available to your colleague when needed. You must be affable. In other words, you should project a sense of wanting to be helpful to your colleague. This raises again the common reaction that many consultant physicians have to certain consult requests as being "bogus" or "inappropriate." These requests may seem that way to you because you have expertise in the area that your colleague doesn't share, but to the colleague requesting your help with a patient he does not fully understand or know how to help, it may seem extremely important and urgent. This is a difficult attitude to master, once again, primarily because of the time pressure you are working under. You may be following 10-20 patients, and you might "triage" your colleague's request for help to a lower level of urgency. But remember, your colleague is worried about this one particular patient, not all the other patients you are caring for. Our job, very simply, is to be helpful to our colleague, regardless of what we may think about the legitimacy of his request. Therefore, the primary attitude that we want to shape is that of <u>availability</u> and <u>affability.</u> The <u>ability</u> attribute will be discussed in the following chapters as we deal with the diagnosis and treatment of specific disorders.

Chapter 3: Organic Brain Disorders

The title of this chapter is conceptually complicated because at some level all psychological disorders are "organic" since there can be no psychological phenomena without a brain to serve as the substrate for psychological functions. The term, "Organic Brain Disorders" has been used as a convenience to describe those brain disorders, associated with psychological symptoms, whose physical pathology has been, to varying degrees, elucidated. It is in this sense that the term is used in this chapter.

The brain is the organ that is the biological substrate for many psychological and somatic functions. Most of these functions can be broadly grouped into two domains, 1) **Sensory-Motor functions**, and, 2) **Psychological (Mental) functions**. The boundaries of these domains are not bright, shining lines, and there is a great deal of overlap, but the boundaries do delineate the areas of interest of the two medical specialties (**Neurology and Psychiatry**) who claim the brain as their area of interest.

Neurology is primarily concerned with pathology of the brain that affects the sensory-motor functions, and psychiatry has, as its primary area of interest, the mental or psychological functions of the brain. As mentioned above, there are many areas of overlap in these domains. Neurology, as a specialty, is becoming increasing interested in disorders of cognition and behavior, and this interest has given rise to the sub-specialty in Neurology of Cognitive-Behavioral Neurology. On the other hand, in the field of **Psychiatry**, there is increased interest in certain motor disorders, such as Catatonia and other complex motor and behavioral disorders which has resulted in the establishment of a subspecialty within Psychiatry called, "Neuro-Psychiatry." These boundaries are constantly shifting, or being gerrymandered, as the two specialties joust for territory. This process is driven by scientific discoveries of how the brain functions. A good example of this is the recent discovery of the auto-immune encephalopathies and the immune-complex pathology that underlies them. The clinical manifestations of these disorders are, initially, psychological (anxiety, confusion, psychosis), but as the auto-immune pathology that underlies these psychological manifestations was more fully characterized, these disorders were claimed by Neurology.

In clinical medicine we are quite used to the concept of organ pathology and its clinical manifestations as "organ failure." It's part of our clinical vocabulary to use terms like "kidney failure" and "heart failure," so it's curious that one rarely, if ever, hears the term "brain failure." This is undoubtedly due to the fact that we know so much less about the functions and dysfunctions of the brain as an organ than we do about the heart, lungs, liver, and kidneys. Nonetheless, the function of the brain, as an organ, does fail, and the resulting state is "Brain Failure."

In this chapter we will discuss the various clinical manifestations of "Brain Failure," and discuss the known or suspected pathological mechanisms that underlie the "Brain Failure." This discussion will be divided into two parts: Clinical manifestations of "Brain Failure" and causes of "Brain Failure."

Clinical Manifestations.

As mentioned in an earlier chapter, it is convenient, though perhaps somewhat reductionistic, to think of all mental (psychological) functions as existing in three domains: **A**ffective/emotional, **B**ehavioral, and **C**ognitive (the "A,B,C's"). Regardless of the validity of this construct, we will use this as a template to organize the discussion of the clinical manifestations of Brain Failure.

Affective/Emotional: Just as there are three primary colors (red, yellow, and blue) that form the basis of all colors and hues, there are five "primary" emotions: happiness, fear, anger, sadness, and shame/guilt. From the mixtures of these five primary emotions come all the richness and nuances of the human emotional spectrum. The subjective experience of an emotion and its expression in affect (facial expression, voice tone, and motor behavior) are modulated by a number of complex neural circuits. When the normal function of these neural circuits is impaired by a pathological process, it can affect how emotions are subjectively experienced and objectively communicated through affect. Although this can occur in many different ways, abnormalities in the function of these emotional circuits usually express themselves in the appropriateness of a particular emotion/affect, the intensity, or volume, of the emotion/affect, and proportionality of the emotion and its expression in affect.

It is perhaps this latter dimension of emotional expression that is most sensitive to pathology affecting these neural circuits. Traditionally, this has been referred to as "Pseudo-Bulbar Palsy." More recently, it has been referred to more graphically as "emotional incontinence" or "Affective Dysregulation Syndrome." Regardless of the term used to denote the condition, there is a disproportionately intense and extreme affective expression resulting from a relatively minor emotional stimulus. This condition is thought to result from pathological processes affecting the higher cortical control and inhibition of sub-cortical (limbic system) neural circuits that constitute the neural substrate of primary emotions. These clinical manifestations are seen in a wide variety of pathological processes that affect the bilateral cerebral cortices. Some of the more common of these conditions are strokes and neuro-degenerative disorders such as Dementia and Parkinson's Disease.

Behavioral Abnormalities: Behavior, like emotion and affect, is controlled by complex processes that mold and shape the contours of behavior. For behavior to be adaptive and effective, it must "fit" the twin demands of internal drives and external reality. To help with this adaptive imperative, the mind (brain) has evolved the ability to self-monitor in real time to determine if the behavior that is manifest is appropriate and to make corrections and adjustments in real time if the behavior is not appropriate to these demands. This complex and finely tuned process is subserved by neural circuits in the Frontal Lobe of the brain. If the function of these circuits is impaired by pathological processes, behavior becomes disordered and dysfunctional.

This is manifested clinically in many ways. The behavior in question may be inappropriate and/or disproportionate. An example of disproportionate behavior is termed "behavioral incontinence" where an extreme and sudden display of anger or sadness occurs in response to a very minor stimulus. The "modulation" of the expression of behavior may be abnormal. The expression, over time, of behavior in response to a stimulus is gradual, much like a light controlled by a "dimmer switch." When this process of modulation is impaired, the expression of behavior over time functions more like a "toggle switch" with a rapid "turn on" and "turn off" of behavior and emotion. Related to this is the ability to modulate and control the "volume" of behavior which can be impaired when pathological processes impair the neural circuits that are responsible for the expression of behavior.

Cognitive Function. As mentioned in Chapter 2 in the discussion of the Mental Status Examination, certain specific cognitive functions can be assessed at the bedside. Pathophysiologic processes affecting brain function will almost invariably affect aspects of cognitive function. Delirium and Dementia are two clinical syndromes that are often seen in the general hospital patient population, and disordered cognition often dominates the clinical picture. These two syndromes (Delirium and Dementia) often overlap in their symptomatic expression. One way to understand the relationship between these two syndromes is to think of a "hierarchy" of cognitive functions. Each cognitive function in this hierarchy is dependent on the functional integrity of the hierarchy is impaired, then all those above it will be impaired. On the other hand, if the functional impairment is higher in the hierarchy, then those cognitive functions below it may be spared and be largely intact. The notion of a "hierarchy" of cognitive functions is a heuristic "model" and is not meant to be taken literally.

Such a hierarchy might look like this:

-Insight and Judgement   -Perception
-Abstract Thinking   -Attention
-Orientation   -Consciousness
-Memory

Delirium is a more global manifestation of "Brain Failure" than is Dementia. The pathophysiological processes involved in Delirium seem to affect those neural circuits (sub-cortical and brainstem) that subserve the functions of consciousness and attention. Since those foundational mental functions are impaired, all those in the hierarchy above it are impaired. This is in contrast with what is typically seen in Dementia, which is a more limited and specific type of Brain Failure than Delirium. In Dementia, it is primarily the cortex and sub-cortical areas that are affected by pathological processes and not the brainstem. This explains why many demented patients may have relatively normal levels of consciousness and may be able to focus attention, but the functions of memory, orientation, abstract thinking, and insight/judgment are impaired. This distinction is an oversimplification of the relationship between Delirium and Dementia. Dementia is known to be a significant risk factor for the development of Delirium, and this explains the phenomenon of Delirium being "layered" over a pre-existing diagnosis of Dementia. When the pathological process affecting those deeper brain circuits subsides, then one may see the appearance of the pre-morbid Dementia. This distinction may help to explain the other differences between Delirium and Dementia. The onset of Delirium is usually acute and tends to fluctuate over a 24-hour period, whereas Dementia comes on gradually and tends to persist with only minor fluctuations. Of most importance, however, is the fact that Delirium is usually reversible whereas Dementia often is not. These distinctions support the notion that the pathological processes and brain circuit dysfunctions for these two disorders may be largely (with some overlap) separate.

ETIOLOGY

In the paragraphs above, there was discussion of the symptomatic and behavioral expression of Organic Brain Disorder. Next we turn to a discussion of the many different causes of these syndromes. This is more than an academic, intellectual exercise for the Consultation Psychiatrist. Consultation Psychiatrists are the experts in the multiple causes of "Brain Failure."

We share this expertise with Neurology, but we must remember that our colleagues in Medicine and Surgery look to us to help them diagnose not just the clinical presentation but what is <u>causing</u> the syndrome. This is crucially important because an understanding of the underlying pathology that produces a clinical picture (subjective symptoms and objective signs) is helpful in choosing the right treatment.

There are many different pathological processes that affect the structure and function of the brain that result in "Brain Failure." In the discussion below, I have tried to organize this by using two mnemonics to aid the clinician in systematically reviewing types of pathological processes that might cause a particular brain syndrome. The first mnemonic is **"VINDICTIVE."** I will very briefly outline the types of pathology involved in each class denoted by the letters in VINDICTIVE, but I will not go into much detail of each pathological process. That exercise would be beyond the scope and purpose of this book.

"V"-VASCULAR

This category includes all vascular and related pathology that affects the blood vessels in the brain that constitutes the supply line or the conduits by which oxygen is delivered to all parts of the brain, particularly those parts in the cortex which are supplied by those vessels with the smallest diameter. Stated simply: neurons love oxygen, and their function is exquisitely sensitive to anything that compromises the supply of oxygen.

The three pathological factors that directly affect the degree to which oxygen is delivered to the brain are:

1) Hemoglobin (the transporter of oxygen).
2) The heart (the pump that pushes the hemoglobin throughout the body).
3) Blood Vessels (the "pipes" through which the blood is pumped).

Any pathological process that affects any one, two, or all three of these factors is going to result in a net deficit of oxygen being delivered to neurons in the brain, and this will compromise the function of those neurons affected. We will focus primarily on the cerebral vasculature in this section. Pathophysiological processes such as Diabetes, Hypertension, or Arteriosclerosis will significantly affect the elasticity and/or the diameter of blood vessels in the brain. The most dramatic example of this is an embolic or hemorrhagic stroke that can deprive the brain of enough oxygen that there is a catastrophic death of neurons with obvious and severe impairment in function. Less drastic examples of pathology affecting cerebral vasculature is small vessel disease of the brain that is often seen in patients who have vascular pathology in other parts of the body (peripheral vascular disease, coronary artery disease). It stands to reason that if a patient has vascular pathology in their heart or peripheral vascular, they almost always will have similar pathology in the brain. These patients are often referred to as "vasculopaths." Also, there are certain inflammatory diseases that affect the cerebral vasculature, such as the Cerebritis/Vasculitis syndromes seen in certain auto-immune diseases like Lupus.

I-INFECTIOUS/INFLAMMATORY

Infection with microbes will produce inflammatory pathology; however, immune complex pathology also involves an inflammatory process. It is the effect of the inflammatory process on neurons, synapses, glia cells, cerebral vasculature, and meninges that can compromise neuronal function and lead to 'brain failure." Also, this causation category (INFECTIOUS/INFLAMMATORY) needs to be conceptually divided into two parts: Those that are intracranial and those that are extracranial.

Intracranial: Among those intracranial infectious processes are bacterial, fungal, protozoal, spirochetal, and viral diseases that directly affect neurons, glial cells, and other intracranial cellular structures. Well known examples of these types of infections are meningitis (bacterial), and encephalitis (HSV) that produce dramatic impairment in brain function resulting brain failure syndromes. HIV infection must also be considered in high risk populations as this virus can also produce a spectrum of clinical syndromes ranging from Dementia to less severe motor-cognitive syndromes. In addition, in the clinical setting of HIV infection, opportunistic infections of the CNS must also be considered. Herpes Simplex Encephalitis, in its early stages, often presents with cognitive and behavioral abnormalities that may mimic closely a functional psychosis.

Extracranial: Infectious and inflammatory processes occurring in other parts of the body may also have effects on the CNS. This effect is a "remote," as opposed to a "direct," effect on the CNS. It has long been noted that patients who have clear evidence of an infection in some part of their body (especially the lower urinary tract) often show signs of cognitive or behavioral abnormality. The mechanism by which this occurred was not known until recently when it was shown that cytokines released into the bloodstream by the peripheral inflammatory process were able to cross the blood-brain barrier into the CNS where they affect neuronal function primarily by adversely affecting neurotransmitter function. This scenario has been supported by other observations from the use of certain cytokines as chemotherapeutic agents in treating viral infections (Hepatitis-C) and malignancies (Renal Cell Carcinoma and Melanoma).

Immune Complex Pathology: There is a rapidly growing body of evidence that shows that antibodies produced in the body in response to various antigens in extracranial tumors cross the Blood-Brain Barrier and affect certain proteins on the neuron, the synapse, or intra-neuronal structures causing severe and significant impairment in neuronal function. It was originally thought that it was only antibodies formed against tumor antigens that caused this problem (para-neoplastic syndromes); however, it appears that this pathology is far more complicated, and that T-Cell mediated factors can also compromise neuronal function. This extremely complicated area of CNS pathology should be thought of as "Auto-Immune Encephalitis," since it is the direct effect on neurons and glia of immune complex pathology that is of crucial importance, regardless of where this immune complex pathology originates.

An additional point of emphasis in this regard is the fact that in the early stages of the evolving pathology of Auto-Immune Encephalitis, the presenting clinical syndrome of this brain pathology is manifest primarily by psychological symptoms of emotional, behavioral, and cognitive abnormalities. Only later in the evolution of the underlying pathology do more classic "neurological" signs (Dysphasia, motor abnormalities, catatonia, and seizures) become manifest.

The above discussion of Infectious/Inflammatory causes of "Brain Failure" is brief, superficial, and incomplete. It is meant only to highlight a broad category of pathological processes that can affect brain function and cause the clinical syndrome of "Brain Failure" (or Delirium/ Dementia) seen at the bedside by the Consultation Psychiatrist.

N-NEOPLASM

Tumors can affect neuronal function, and this can occur with both intracranial tumors and extracranial tumors. It is easy to understand how certain intracranial tumors can affect brain function by exerting a mass effect on neurons and neural circuits that support certain sensory, motor, and higher cortical functions. It is, perhaps, less intuitively understood how extracranial tumors can affect brain function.

This occurs by way of the para-neoplastic process mentioned above in the discussion of auto-immune encephalitis. To briefly reprise this discussion, antibodies are formed against cell surface proteins on certain tumors, e.g., small cell lung cancer, germ cell tumors (teratomas), ovarian and testicular tumors, and thymomas. These antibodies react against similar antigens on certain neurons producing immune complex pathology that impairs neuronal function. Depending on the neural circuits affected by this immune complex pathology, brain function impairment may be expressed as a sensory, motor, or psychological deficit.

D-DEGENERATIVE

This is a broad category of many different types of neuropathology that share a common pathological denominator of slow, chronic, and progressive degeneration of nerve tissue that, depending on the number and type of neurons affected, may significantly affect brain function. The prototypic disease that exemplifies this category is Alzheimer's Disease, but there are other degenerative diseases such as Fronto-Temporal Dementia, Lewy Body Dementia, Huntington's Disease, and Parkinson's Disease. These degenerative diseases usually produce a clinical syndrome characterized by Dementia with specific cognitive deficits in abstract thinking, speech, memory, and orientation that dominate the overall clinical picture.

It is important to remember that Dementia is the single most important "risk factor" for the development of a Delirium. The slow, indolent progression of a degenerative brain process may go unnoticed or under-appreciated until the development of a superimposed delirium. Once the delirium clears, one may see the underlining Dementia.

I-INTERVENTRICULAR

This category of pathology includes all those pathological processes that affect CSF circulation and pressure dynamics. One such example is "Normal Pressure Hydrocephalus" (NPH). This is not a common disorder, but it should be considered in any differential diagnosis of Brain Failure since, in certain selected cases, neurosurgical intervention may have significant therapeutic benefit.

A clinical "triad" of dementia, urinary incontinence, and gait disturbance is often associated with NPH, and the presence of this clinical "triad" might increase the diagnostic yield of brain imaging studies to make this diagnosis.

C-CONGENITAL

This category includes a large number of neuropathological states caused by genetic abnormalities, prenatal, and perinatal abnormalities. Cerebral Palsy is one specific example of this class of disorders. Other examples are: Fetal Alcohol Syndrome, Fragile X Syndrome, and the large number of inborn errors of metabolism that may be clinically manifest as Brain Failure.

As a convenience to the integrity of the VINDICTIVE mnemonic, we also include in this category Seizure Disorders, although many seizure disorders are not due to congenital pathological processes. Seizure Disorders are common, however, and it should be remembered that throughout the natural course of seizure disorders, psychological symptoms and signs (**A-B-C**'s) may be among the broad array of the clinical picture of seizure disorders.

There are <u>four</u> compartments or stages that constitute the natural history of a seizure, and each stage can manifest abnormal psychological phenomena:

1) **Aura.** This stage can be manifest as symptoms of dissociative phenomena (e.g., feelings of depersonalization and derealization).

2) **Ictal** event. Although we usually think of an actual seizure event as characterized primarily by dramatic motor signs such as a grand mal, or major motor seizure, the seizure event may be characterized primarily by abnormal cognition and/or behavior as seen, for instance, in a Temporal Lobe Seizure or Frontal Lobe seizures.

3) **Post-Ictal** state. This state immediately following the termination of the seizure is often characterized by abnormal cognition (decreased level of consciousness, disorientation) and agitated behavior.

4) **Inter-Ictal** states. There is a growing body of evidence pointing to abnormal brain functioning occurring between seizures (ictal events). This may be manifest by abnormal mood states, periods of dissociative phenomena, and psychotic symptoms. Personality traits that are thought to be specific to patients with epilepsy have been attributed to "inter-ictal" pathology. These traits are hyper-religiosity with intense spiritual experiences, a tendency to compulsively write about one's personal experiences, and increases and decreases in sexual feelings and behavior.

It is difficult to know how specific these traits are to people with epilepsy. One epileptologist. Eli Goldensohn, coined a beautifully vivid metaphor to describe this process. He called it the "burning ember" model. In this metaphor, the seizure focus functions much like a burning ember in a bed of coals. A whiff of oxygen will cause the glowing ember to burst into flames, and this is analogous to the seizure focus causing an ictal event (seizure). But while the ember is just glowing (quiescent), it is still radiating considerable amounts of heat and light in the immediate surroundings, just as a seizure focus (a neuropathological process) is still exerting some pathological effect on the neural tissue immediately surrounding the actual seizure focus. Depending on the location of the glowing "ember" (seizure focus), this pathology might be expressed clinically in inter-ictal sensory and cognitive phenomena that may be perceived by the patient.

T-TRAUMA

It is obvious that physical trauma can adversely affect any biological tissue by the transmission of sufficient kinetic energy to disrupt the structural and functional integrity of tissue. This is clearly no less evident in the case of trauma to the brain. Pathological causes of Brain Failure can occur as a result of closed head trauma or direct injury to brain tissue as a result of surgical or blunt force trauma. Other examples of pathology that directly affect the structure of neurons and neuronal circuits are contusions, shearing injury as a result of rapid acceleration-deceleration of the brain inside the calvarium, subdural and epidural hematomas, and diffuse or localized cerebral edema. Recently, there has been a lot of much needed attention on the post-concussion syndrome which has both acute and chronic symptoms of Brain Failure.

I-INTOXICATION/WITHDRAWAL

This category includes all exogenous substances that may adversely affect brain function. This class of pathology is perhaps the single most common cause of Brain Failure, and it should be at the top of the list for every physician who attempts to investigate causes of Brain Failure. Two other considerations about this group of causes must be remembered. 1. It is the least expensive to diagnose, but remember to ask about it and take a careful history, or order a urine drug screen, and, 2. Once identified, the toxic substance can usually be removed, thus insuring some degree of reversibility of Brain Failure.

There are five groups of potentially toxic substances that should be considered as possible causes of Brain Failure:

Illicit Drugs. This group includes drugs such as alcohol, stimulants, sedatives, narcotics, and hallucinogens that are usually taken for recreational or psychological reasons. The toxic and withdrawal effects are well known, and they will not be detailed here. A more detailed description and discussion of treatment will be found in the chapter devoted to Substance Use Disorders.

Medically Prescribed Drugs. Many drugs prescribed by physicians for non-CNS conditions may have secondary and unintended effects on brain function. Some common examples are opiate analgesics, corticosteroids, immunosuppressants, antihistamines, antispasmodics, and anti-parkinsonian drugs, to name just a few. This is another inexpensive diagnostic endeavor. All you need to do is just remember to think of it and take a careful history of the medications that a patient is taking.

Over-The-Counter Medications. (OTC) This group of substances is often referred to as the "Hidden Pharmacopea." Most physicians never think to ask what O-T-C medications a patient may be taking, and most patients don't mention these medications to their doctors when asked under the assumption that non-prescription substance are not that clinically significant. Many O-T-C medications such as sleep aids, cold remedies, and stimulants have well established effects on the CNS. The magnitude of the "Hidden Pharmacopea" can be appreciated by any visit to a supermarket or pharmacy. Huge amounts of shelf space are devoted to stocking these substances. Any retailer will tell you that there is a direct and powerful correlation between consumer demand and amount of shelf space. A lot of your patients may be taking some of these OTC preparations, and it's important to ask about them.

Herbal and Mineral Supplements. Over the past decade there has been a virtual explosion in the number of people who feel they can enhance their health and performance and protect against illness by taking some preparation that usually contains various naturally occurring ingredients. Some have direct CNS effects (e.g., Valerian) and others have indirect effects (e.g., St. John's Wort). Most of these substances are ineffective and harmless, but some may have clinically significant effects either directly or indirectly by affecting metabolizing enzymes in the liver that may affect levels of other drugs. An example of one such clinically significant interaction is St. John's Wort taken in conjunction with immunosuppressants. The St. John's Wort induces the metabolism of many immunosuppressants, and this results in lower blood levels of the immunosuppressants that puts the post-transplant patient at risk for graft rejection.

Environmental Toxins. This category includes heavy metals, exposure to pesticides, carbon monoxide, and organic solvents that adversely affect brain function. It is important to ask about possible exposure to these substances.

V-VITAMIN DEFICIENCIES

Deficiencies of one or more vitamins may affect neuronal function and, secondarily, cause varying degrees of Brain Failure. This is particularly the case with deficiency of thiamine, niacin, folate, and B-12. The most notable example of the interaction of vitamin deficiency and abnormal neuronal function is seen in the case of thiamine deficiency and the resulting clinical syndromes of Wernicke's Encephalopathy and Korsakoff's Syndrome. The causes of vitamin deficiency are related to inadequate dietary intake of foods containing essential vitamins and/or poor absorption in the small intestine where most vitamins are absorbed. Patients with poor dietary intake secondary to psychological factors (e.g., Anorexia Nervosa, Alcoholism) or chronic systemic illness should be considered at risk for these conditions. In addition, patients with intrinsic GI pathology (e.g., alcoholism, Inflammatory Bowel Disease) may not absorb sufficient vitamins. Decreased absorption of certain vitamins must always be considered in patients who have had bariatric surgery for Morbid Obesity.

E-ENDOCRINE/METABOLIC

Endocrine. Various endocrine disorders can affect CNS function. In considering this category of possible causes of Brain Failure, start anatomically from top to bottom. Pituitary and Hypothalamic dysfunction can indirectly affect brain function through its effect on other endocrine systems. Next is thyroid dysfunction, and both increases and decreases in thyroid hormone production can cause CNS dysfunction. Para-Thyroid dysfunction can result in changes in brain function through its effect on abnormal levels of serum calcium. Pancreas gland (islet cells) dysfunction, by causing elevated or decreased levels of blood sugar, can affect brain function. Finally, Adrenal gland pathology (either hypo or hyper-function) can produce clinical syndromes (Addison's Disease or Cushing's Syndrome) with prominent psychological symptomatology. Patients with Addison's Disease usually have profound fatigue and depression, and patients with Cushing's Disease may exhibit signs of hypomania or mania.

Metabolic. Pathological states involving the lungs, heart, liver, and kidneys can produce metabolic changes that adversely affect brain function. In regard to pathology involving the lungs and/or the heart resulting in decreased oxygen being absorbed (lungs) or pumped (heart), we are reminded that neurons are exquisitely sensitive to decreases in oxygen and sugar. Any pathological state resulting in decreases in oxygen and/or sugar will quickly and directly affect neuronal function. One of the many functions of the liver is to metabolize and detoxify certain substances. One example of this is the detoxification of CNS-active polypeptides that are absorbed from the GI tract. In certain cases of liver dysfunction, this ability is impaired with the resulting accumulation of these CNS active polypeptides. One of these proteins is ammonia which, when elevated, can dramatically affect brain function producing Hepatic Encephalopathy. Although rare, one must also think of other hepatic causes of Brain Failure such as Wilson's Disease and Porphyria. Kidney failure can affect brain function either by decreases in glomerular filtration resulting in increase in BUN and Creatinine or by causing electrolyte abnormalities such as hyponatremia or hypernatremia.

The conditions listed, and briefly described, above in the **VINDICTIVE** mnemonic format comprise most of the causes of Brain Failure. Since Brain Failure is such a potentially devastating pathological entity, it is important that you have some method of systematically reviewing the causes of this condition so you can suggest to the patient's physician how to embark on a diagnostic process and treat the underlying pathological cause(s) of Brain Failure. I have had numerous trainees in Consultation Psychiatry defer to internists or neurologists to do the "Dementia Workup." This is a mistake. The Psychiatrist, and particularly, the Consultation Psychiatrist, is the expert in diagnosing and treating Brain Failure in the same way that a cardiologist is the expert in cardiac failure and the hepatologist is the expert in hepatic failure, and so on with each organ. It is true that we share the expertise in Brain Failure with neurologists, but in my experience even this expertise may be highly variable among neurologists.

There is one major problem with the **VINDICTIVE** mnemonic, and that is the fact that it is overly comprehensive. It takes a long time to think through all the possibilities encompassed in the mnemonic and to embark on the diagnostic process to run them down, not to mention the extremely expensive nature of such a comprehensive Brain Failure workup. Most of the pathological entities included in that mnemonic are uncommon. In clinical situations like this there needs to be a "screen" that focuses on those pathological conditions that most often cause Brain Failure. This allows you to target your efforts more effectively and efficiently.

A clinically useful screen that has been helpful in our hands involves yet another mnemonic: "**OMIT.**" This can be remembered by the saying to yourself, "never omit, **OMIT**" when evaluating a patient with Brain Failure. Like all such mnemonics, each letter stands for something you need to think of in these circumstances.

"O"-Oxygen.

It is axiomatic that neurons require oxygen in order to function. Every medical student has learned about the high (relative to other cells and tissues in the body) oxygen requirements unique to neurons. Therefore, any condition that results in a net decrease, or partial or permanent absence, of oxygen to neurons will significantly affect brain function. There are three obvious variables that affect the amount of oxygen transported to the brain:

- The transporters of oxygen (hemoglobin)
- The pump (heart) that propels the "carriers" to the brain
- The diameter and integrity of the vessels through which the blood is pumped.

Any pathological condition that affects any one or more of these three variables will have a net effect of decreasing oxygen to the cells that are the "hungriest" for it. Without sufficient oxygen, quite simply the brain starts to fail.

"M"- Metabolic

Neurons can only function normally within a fairly narrow range of perturbations of the metabolic milieu. The metabolic milieu is composed of many elements, but it is primarily the ionic, osmotic, and toxic (NH_3 and centrally active polypeptides and monoamines, BUN, oxidative radicals, and others) environment that directly affects neuronal function. The kidney, liver, and, to some extent, the lungs are the organs that regulate these metabolic products. When these organs fail, the metabolic sequelae of this failure will affect neuronal function. Therefore, under the "M" of the OMIT mnemonic, one should look at Liver Function Tests (particularly NH_3) and check levels of electrolytes (including Ca and Mg).

"I"- INFECTIOUS/INFLAMMATORY

Clinicians have long noted the association of infectious and inflammatory pathological processes with signs of Delirium, but the causal mechanisms were not clear. Research over the past decade has elucidated some of these mechanisms, and it appears as though components of the inflammatory cascade (particularly cytokines) are able to pass through the Blood Brain Barrier and, once in the CNS, can have significant effects on neuronal function. One effect of cytokines in the brain is to alter serotonin metabolism by shunting Tryptophan to an alternative pathway to the production of Kynurenin. This results in less tryptophan available to synthesize serotonin. In thinking about this class of causes of brain failure, we must avoid the pitfall of focusing solely on the wide variety (bacterial, viral, fungal, parasitic, and others) of infections by microbial agents. Remember that this class of causes includes "inflammatory" causes that may be immune mediated in the absence of an acute microbial infection. A primary example of this are the Auto-Immune Encephalopathies described above.

"T"-TOXIC

This category in the **OMIT** mnemonic includes primarily exogenous toxins that have CNS effects. It is important to think of three subcategories of toxins: prescribed medications, illicit or recreational toxins, and Over-The-Counter (OTC) substances. The latter two categories have often been described as the "hidden pharmacopeia" because they are widely used substances but, because they are not "prescribed" by physicians we rarely ask about them.

1. Prescribed medications with CNS effects: There are a large number of medications prescribed by physicians that have un-intended effects on CNS function. Some of the most common of these are:

   - Opiates
   - Anti-Cholinergics: anti-histamines, anti-spasmodics for GI and GU disorders, bronchodilators, and mydriatics.
   - Antibiotics: Quinilones.

- Dopamine agonists, e.g., treatment for patients with Parkinson's Syndrome) and Dopamine antagonists (GI drugs pro-kinetics).

2. Illicit and recreational drugs are taken for the specific purpose of altering CNS function. Always ask about their use (especially if your patient is a doctor!)

3. OTC and Dietary Supplements. A marketing maxim states that the amount of shelf space featuring a product(s) is in direct proportion to the demand for these products. This speaks to the wide use of these products in our society. Many of these products contain substances that affect CNS function, e.g., cold remedies, sleep aids, antispasmodics, in addition to those substances targeted directly at psychological symptoms, e.g., St. John's Wort, Valerian, and others.

In summary, the **OMIT** mnemonic will help you to focus on a sub-set of causes of brain failure with a much higher diagnostic yield at lower cost in terms of your time and cost to the health care "treasury." In my clinical experience, the use of the OMIT mnemonic as a screen has a yield of @85% of the causes of Brain Failure.

MOLECULAR/CELLULAR FACTORS

The categories of pathophysiological causes discussed above have what might be termed a final common pathway of cellular metabolic perturbation that is the proximate cause of Brain Failure. Not a lot is known about the cellular pathology that is responsible for the neuronal dysfunction underlying Brain Failure, but it can be conceptualized as operating on three system levels, each in increasing order of complexity. The first level is what occurs intracellularly and at the receptor. The second level is what occurs with organized aggregates of neurons that we call "neuronal circuits."

The third and most complex system is at the level of Brain function which integrates the function of numerous neuronal circuits and expresses itself in psychological phenomena (emotion, behavior, and cognition). Most of the causes of brain failure discussed above have their final common pathway at the cellular (neuronal level) and are characterized by "oxidative stress" resulting in calcium influx which affects mitochondrial function. This, in turn, has an effect on neurotransmitter function at the pre and post synaptic receptors.

Two neurotransmitters, Dopamine and Acetylcholine, are thought to be particularly important in the cellular pathophysiology underlying Brain Failure. Any perturbation that results in increasing dopaminergic tone or decreasing cholinergic tone is thought to be critical in this process. It is certainly overly simplistic to think that these are the only neurotransmitters that play a role in Delirium. There is evidence that glutamate (NMDA), which is the major excitatory transmitter, and GABA, the major inhibitory transmitter, also plays an important role. For a more detailed discussion of this complex intracellular process that underlies the clinical syndrome of Delirium, see the excellent discussion by Fricchione *et al* in (Am. J. Psychiat. 165: 7, July, 2008, p. 803-812).

DYNAMIC INTERACTION OF CAUSATIVE FACTORS

It is perhaps stating the obvious to say that the brain is a highly dynamic biologic system; nonetheless, I will state it here for emphasis. The past few sections of this chapter have focused on pathophysiological causes of Brain Failure. Stating and listing these causes creates a type of cognitive artifact in how we think about the interactions of these causes in such a highly dynamic system. We think of them as a type of "freeze frame" in what is really a constantly changing interaction over time. Heraclitus' famous statement that a man can never step twice in the same place in a river is an illustration of this point. One individual can experience a "hit" to the brain at age 20 and experience the same "hit" forty years later at age 60, and the symptomatic expression of these "hits" might be quite different.

This is illustrated in Figure 3.1.

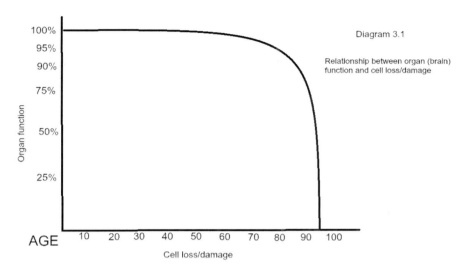

Diagram 3.1

Relationship between organ (brain) function and cell loss/damage

The "y" axis represents organ function (in this case, brain function), but it can apply equally well to the function of other organs, e.g., heart, kidneys, lungs, or liver. The "x" axis represents time and the accumulated "burden" over time of cell loss due to normal ageing or pathological "hits" to the cells in brain. Age can be viewed as a "proxy" for cell damage and loss, but one can experience brain cell damage/loss at any age and this would "push" the patient further to the right along the "x" axis. The point to emphasize here is that a sodium of 120 Meq/L at age 30 in a person who has a normal brain will have a very different effect on function that the same sodium level of 120 Meq/L in a person of 80. As one progresses to the right on the "x" axis, the curve transitions from showing incremental change to showing exponential change.

An additional point to be made in this context has to do with the way physicians are trained to think. We are trained to use the Law of Parsimony or "Occam's Razor" when thinking about the causes of illness. In other words, we try to explain an illness presentation with one diagnosis or one pathological cause.

Sir William Osler issued a cautionary note on this issue with his aphorism, "A man can have both lice and fleas." We need to remember that there may be <u>more than one cause</u> for a particular clinical syndrome. This is particularly the case in Brain Failure.

The basic message here is that nature (and biology) are not simple. It is messy, complex, and constantly changing. It is very important to remember this when attempting to figure out what is causing the Brain Failure of the patient you are examining.

THE DIAGNOSTIC PROCESS

To repeat what was mentioned earlier in this chapter, the job of the consultation psychiatrist in evaluating a patient with Brain Failure is threefold:

1) to make the clinical diagnosis at the bedside.
2) to recommend treatment for the patient.
3) to search for a cause (or causes) of the Brain Failure.

The diagnostic process can be complicated, arduous (for the patient), and potentially very expensive. Responsible physicians must be aware of their duty to be thoughtful stewards of the economic health care enterprise, and not needlessly waste resources on expensive, but low-yield diagnostic testing. Quite appropriately, much has been made of the extremely high cost of medical care that, unless contained, threatens to bankrupt the health care enterprise in this country. One component of health care costs is the cost of diagnostic testing.

There are two overarching reasons why diagnostic testing costs so much: The first is that we have such incredible diagnostic technology that enables us to know so much, and it is natural that we would want to employ this wonderful technology in the service of our patients. The second factor is a unique peculiarity of our health care economy, and that is the disconnect from the behavior of "buying" diagnostic tests and the cost of these tests. Intellectually we know that nothing is free in this world, but when we sit in front of a computer in a nurses' station to enter orders for diagnostic tests, some of which may costs thousands of dollars, we are not conscious of how much they cost. We just order them.

This often takes the form of "pan-testing" where we might order every conceivable test (including very expensive brain imaging) as part of a diagnostic fishing expedition hoping to catch something. The medical culture in which we live and work unwittingly reinforces this behavior. We hate to "miss something," so we cover all our bases. As an example of how we are taught to do this, remember how many times in our training we were asked by our teachers, "why didn't you order a...," rather than, "Why did you order that...."? Numerous professional societies have stated that "unnecessary care" or wastefulness (including diagnostic testing) constitutes as much as a third of all health care expenses. So unnecessary test ordering constitutes a major problem, and it behooves us to be very thoughtful about how we go about this.

There are two "rules of thumb" that help guide us in thoughtful test ordering: 1. Ask yourself if the result of the test will clearly affect treatment intervention, and, 2. In suspected cases of rare disorders, e.g., Folate or B-12 deficiency causing Brain Failure, ask yourself if there are screening procedures which would increase the likelihood of a positive yield, e.g., checking a CBC or testing the patient for posterior column disease in the case of suspected Folate/B-12 deficiency.

TREATMENT

Often we need to institute symptomatic treatment of the delirious patient before we have an etiological diagnosis. The conceptual foundation for this approach involves an understanding of the neuronal pathophysiology outlined above. Our pharmacologic treatment of delirium primarily targets receptors, usually dopamine receptors. It is possible that other receptors might be suitable targets for treatment of delirium such as serotonin and glutamate-NMDA receptors, and voltage gated cation channels that act on axonal membranes and not receptors; however, we usually use neuroleptics, that act as dopamine antagonists, as first line treatments. There is no standard dosage of neuroleptics, but most follow a "start low, go slow" practice since most patients with Brain Failure are usually medically compromised and will be less able to tolerate side effects.

All standard neuroleptics have been tried in the treatment of Delirium, and there is evidence to support the effectiveness of all of them. What is lacking, however, are comparative effectiveness trials to help us select one or another neuroleptic that is more effective than the other or has fewer side effects. Standard practice favors dividing the daily dose of neuroleptic into two doses with 2/3 of the total daily dose given as an HS dose since Delirium seems to increase at night.

Delirium (Brain Failure) is an extremely serious condition, and this fact requires the consultation psychiatrist to see the patient every day (or more frequently) to evaluate the effectiveness of treatment and to make dosage adjustments as needed. Once the patient's symptoms respond, then it is equally important to continue following the patient to decrease and discontinue, if possible, the neuroleptic before the patient is discharged. In the current hospital culture patients are discharged as quickly as possible, and they are often transitioned to a lower level of care where psychiatric care may not be available. In this case, it is absolutely necessary to arrange for outpatient follow up if the patient is still on neuroleptics since most physicians are very reluctant to discontinue a neuroleptic that has been started by someone else during a hospitalization. For this reason, many patients have remained on neuroleptics for months, and even years, long after their delirium has cleared. This issue is clinically problematic following the numerous studies that have shown an increase in mortality in demented patients who are maintained on neuroleptics chronically.

Make it a "rule of thumb" that if a patient is discharged before the neuroleptic has been tapered and discontinued the patient must have psychiatric follow up on an outpatient basis. For further discussion of the use of neuroleptics in the medical population, see the chapter on "Pharmacology in the Medically Ill."

Chapter 4: Somatic Symptom Disorders

There is nothing more fascinating than the human mind. This is a truism, and it's the reason many of us have chosen to enter the field of Psychiatry. There are many fascinating things about the mind, but I submit that one of the most interesting things is the tendency, in certain individuals and under various circumstances, to form the subjective experience of being physically ill when there is no objective evidence of pathophysiology that would explain this subjective experience.

To properly explain this further it is necessary to appreciate the distinction between the terms, <u>illness</u> and <u>disease</u>. As physicians we often use these terms interchangeably and incorrectly. <u>Illness</u> is the subjective experience of being sick or experiencing malaise. Illness has cognitive, emotional, and physical dimensions. <u>Disease</u>, on the other hand, is the objective phenomena of physical pathology. Doctors see disease in an x-ray, or abnormal lab values, or on physical examination. Illness is something that is felt or experienced by the patient. Illness not seen. Doctors see, feel, and treat disease. Disease is something that is objectively verifiable. Patients experience illness as a purely subjective experience that has no objective correlates. When we look at an EKG or coronary arteriogram, we say the patient has cardiac "disease," not cardiac "illness." On the other hand, if I am the person with cardiac disease, I do not say, "I have cardiac "illness"; I say, "I have cardiac 'disease.'" I might say, I feel "ill" because I have cardiac "disease." With most patients who have "disease," the subjective experience of illness is proportionate to the extent of disease. If one of these constructs (illness or disease) is disproportionate to the other, it becomes highly maladaptive. There are two examples to illustrate this important distinction.

Disease without illness. This occurs when a patient has serious pathology (disease) but is minimally aware of it, does not feel particularly ill, or behaves as though he is not sick (disease). This is sometimes seen in patients who utilize the defense mechanism of denial in a maladaptive way. They may know that they are sick and may even feel ill, but with the defense mechanism of denial this is minimized in their subjective experience. The obvious problem here is that they may postpone seeing a doctor and getting properly diagnosed and treated. This type of medical denial may be a cause of clinically significant non-compliance with treatment.

Illness without Disease. This occurs when the patient experiences the feeling of illness and behaves as an ill person would behave (decreased function, care seeking behavior, etc.) when there is little or no objective evidence of physical pathology that would explain the degree of subjective malaise (illness) and decreased function. It is this group of patients (those with illness without disease) that forms the population of people that are thought to have a Somatic Symptom Disorder. Later in this chapter we will discuss a new physiological model, that has recently been introduced, that explains these "non-physiologic/non-anatomic" somatic perceptions on the basis of neuro-physiologic mechanism rather than psychological mechanisms.

Terminology
These clinical syndromes have been called many different things over the decades (and centuries). Many of the diagnoses and terms related to these syndromes overlap with one another, and some of them (conversion disorder, in particular) are burdened by reference to the putative psychodynamic causes of the disorder. Examples of the variety of names and terms are: Neurasthenia, Conversion, Somatizing Disorders, Somatoform Disorders, Hypochondriasis, Somatic Delusions, and, more recently, Medically Unexplained Physical Symptoms or Medically Unexplained Somatic Symptoms (MUPS or MUSS). All these terms have had their time in the limelight of popular and professional usage, but then they slowly fade as they are replaced by other terms.

The most recent iteration of this process is the latest DSM-V nomenclature that lumps these entities under one rubric, "Somatic Symptomatic Disorder." In doing this, however, DSM-V has significantly widened the scope of this diagnostic category to include patients who have known, objectively verifiable pathology underlying their sensory somatic symptoms, but who have an abnormal or disproportionate emotional or behavioral response to their illness. Using the "Disease/Illness" dichotomy described above, these are patients who have obvious disease, but their illness is significantly disproportionate to the type and extent of their disease.

The diagnostic terms described briefly above are abstract constructs. They comprise groupings of signs and symptoms in addition to other factors such as history (duration) and effect on function. Problems arise when these terms are reified and lose whatever construct validity they might possess. It is clinically helpful to think about these disorders at a lower level of abstraction in terms of the specific symptoms (and occasionally signs) that patients experience. Listed below, and grouped under organ systems, are most of the common (and some uncommon) syndromes in which patients experience sensory somatic symptoms without clear, or sufficient, evidence of physical pathology that explains them.

CNS:

- Headache
- Dizziness
- Chronic Widespread Pain/Chronic Regional Pain Syndrome
- Phantom Limb Pain
- Charles Bonnet Syndrome
- Chronic Fatigue Syndrome
- Chemical (Environmental) Sensitivity Syndrome
- Gulf War Syndrome
- Agent Orange Syndrome
- Silicone Breast Implant Syndrome

Cardio-Vascular:

- Non-Cardiac Chest Pain
- Phantom Defibrillator Shock Syndrome
- POTS

Gastro-Intestinal:

- Cyclical Vomiting Syndrome
- Irritable Bowel Syndrome
- Globus Dysphagia
- Burning Mouth Syndrome
- Gluten Sensitivity

Respiratory:

- Suffocation (non-physiologic air hunger) Syndrome

Musculoskeletal:

- Temperomandibular Joint Syndrome
- Whiplash
- Chronic Low Back Pain Syndrome

GU:

- Interstitial Cystitis
- Vestibulitis/Vulvodynia
- Chronic Pelvic Pain

Derm:

- Central Itch Syndrome.
- Burning Scrotum Syndrome.
- Morgellons/Parasitosis.

This list of organ based syndromes is how most patients present to their primary care providers (PCP), and these are some of the descriptive names (diagnoses) that are applied to them. The basic defining characteristic of all of them, however, is a grouping of sensory somatic symptoms that have either no, or insufficient, objective evidence of pathology that explains them.

Epidemiology. These somatic symptom disorders are extremely common (Fink et al: Psychosomatics; 1999, 40:330-338). This statement is not surprising to most PCPs since they are the ones who see and follow these patients. This is surprising, however, to most psychiatrists because they rarely see these patients in psychiatric emergency rooms, psychiatric in-patient units, clinics, or outpatient offices. From an epidemiologic perspective, however, they constitute by far the most common type of psychiatric disorder, far more common than any other single psychiatric diagnostic group. Some examples of the epidemiologic data that support this statement is the study by Escobar (Annals of Family Medicine; 2007, vol 5:328-334.) who found in a community sample a prevalence of 4-20%. The simple point here is that there are large numbers of these patients, and most of them are never seen by psychiatrists.

Cost: Another important point to keep in mind when thinking about this group of patients is that they impose a significant cost to the health care "treasury" that is disproportionate to their numbers. Many of these patients are known as "high utilizers" of health care, and the problem is that their high utilization of health care resources does not add value to their health and function. Their "high utilization" status occurs because they make more frequent visits to their PCPs; they have more diagnostic studies; they have a higher rate of referrals to specialists because their symptoms are often confusing; they have more and longer duration in-patient admissions.

The important point here is that there are a lot of these patients and they are costly. This is all the more reason why we need to know about them and know how to help them.

COMMON SOMATIC SYNDROMES
What we call things is important, but it can also be confusing at times. If we lump into one group all patients who have somatic symptoms without demonstrable or sufficient evidence of organic pathology (illness without disease), we will have a very large but very heterogenous group. An analogy that illustrates this point is to lump all patients with anemia into one group. The members of this group would have only one thing in common: an abnormally low hemoglobin, but they would be quite

different in terms of etiology, response to treatments, and co-morbid disorders. It is much the same with patients who have these types of somatic disorders. They differ in regard to the organ systems involved, co-occurring psychiatric symptoms, psychodynamic theories of causation (e.g., Conversion D/O), and a number of other factors. The categories described below are arbitrary, but they have been in use for a while, so we will use some of them in this section; however, keep in mind that the "diagnostic deck" can and will be "reshuffled" in the future, and the diagnostic categories may be different from the way they are now.

SECONDARY SOMATIC SYNDROMES

The defining characteristic of this group is that it contains patients who have somatic symptoms that are clearly secondary to an underlying primary psychiatric disorder.

Depression: Some patients with a clear Depressive D/O may have somatic symptoms along with the usual psychological symptoms that we ordinarily associate with Depression, e.g., sad mood, hopelessness, loss of interest. Depressed patients may de-emphasize these psychological symptoms and emphasize somatic symptoms such as diffuse pain, headache, fatigue, nausea, dizziness. When the Depression is successfully treated, the somatic symptoms often disappear.

Schizophrenia: Certain patients with schizophrenia may present with bizarre somatic symptoms that tend to clearly dominate the clinical picture. These somatic symptoms may initially eclipse the usual positive and negative psychological symptoms that we associate with schizophrenia.

This is illustrated by the clinical vignette that follows.

An undergraduate student presented to the Emergency Room complaining of severe RUQ abdominal pain. He was admitted to the Medical Service for further evaluation. An exhaustive diagnostic workup revealed no objective evidence of organic pathology that would explain the pain. The student remained curled up in the fetal position complaining of continued pain, but he was able to eat and drink normally. The medical resident thought there was something "weird" about the patient and requested a psychiatry consultation. The psychiatry resident and attending interviewed the patient together. The resident asked the patient to describe the pain, and the patient answered, "My pain feels like I have the chopped off head of a rooster with a razor sharp beak that is slicing up my liver into microtome thin slices."

While the resident was asking questions, the attending was looking around the patient's hospital room, and he noticed a textbook that was open on the bedside stand (it was final exam time, and the student had brought with him some books to study). After leaving the room, the attending mentioned the book on the bedside table. It was a book of Greek mythology that the patient was studying for his Classics exam. The book was opened to a well-known myth, and there was an illustration of a famous painting by Rubens showing an eagle eating the liver of a Greek god, Prometheus. This seemed like more than a coincidence, and they went back to the patient and asked him about his understanding of the Prometheus myth. He then explained that he was Prometheus, and the eagle had somehow transformed itself into a rooster that was eating his liver. He also described auditory hallucination of other Greek gods who were talking to him. The patient's abdominal pain was due to the eagle (i.e., the rooster with the razor-sharp beak) eating his liver.

The point here is that this patient was obviously psychotic (delusional and experiencing auditory hallucinations), but this was not appreciated initially because somatic symptoms dominated the clinical picture. It is an example of somatic symptoms (admittedly bizarre) being secondary to a primary, underlying psychiatric disorder.

Anxiety. Patients with anxiety often experience and express their anxiety in somatic terms. This is largely due to the many neuronal circuits that connect the amygdala and limbic area structures with the hypothalamus and the autonomic nervous system. Patients with anxiety (and particularly panic symptoms) often present initially to non-psychiatric physicians because their somatic symptoms so dominate the clinical picture that they eclipse the underlying, defining emotional component of anxiety/panic. Anyone who has worked in an emergency room setting is familiar with the picture of a patient who is rushed by ambulance with symptoms of severe air-hunger, chest pain, and diaphoresis. For obvious reasons an acute cardio-respiratory event must be ruled out. Often aggressive diagnostic testing fails to reveal any objective signs of physical pathology. On careful questioning, the history of anxiety or panic is developed, and that explains the dramatic somatic presentation. The somatic symptoms in this scenario are secondary to an underlying psychological disorder (e.g., anxiety or panic).

Malingering. It is important to be very careful in making this diagnosis and attaching this label to a patient because, if inaccurate, it can be very hurtful to the patient. Once this word (malingering) gets attached to a patient, it "trails" the patient throughout their life (especially in the age of electronic medical records), and it negatively biases future physicians who encounters the patient causing them to view any future complaint through this negative lens.

Malingering means something quite specific. It refers to a person who intentionally and consciously feigns physical symptoms and signs for the purpose of achieving some form of secondary gain. The secondary gain may be positive or negative. Positive secondary gain refers to the desire to have something that is valued like money, drugs, or sympathy from others. Negative secondary gain is the avoidance of something that is perceived to be painful or uncomfortable or upsetting. An example would be a person who feigns a physical symptom to avoid having to attend school or work or prison.

The key issue here is that the secondary gain (positive or negative) is understandable and plausible, although the conscious <u>deception</u> involved in achieving the secondary gain is what gives the whole process its negative moral value. An analogy that captures the essence of the psychological process (though not the moral aspect) involved in malingering is the artistic endeavor of <u>acting</u>. The accomplished actor/actress uses his powers of "deception" to fool the audience into thinking that he is someone he really is not, (e.g., King Lear), and he does so for "secondary gain," in this case the applause, esteem of the audience, and a paycheck for his efforts. But the audience knows before the encounter with the actor that he will attempt to deceive the audience, and the audience attends the performance in the hopes of a really good deception. The actor intentionally and consciously sets out to deceive the audience, and he hopes his behavior will result in secondary gain. In this way, we might think of a malingerer as a "medical thespian" who consciously and intentionally sets out to act the role of a person who is sick in the hopes of deceiving the audience, (e.g., his physician or a disability board), with the motivation of receiving some secondary gain. The difference between the actor and the malingerer is in the" audience"; the theatre-goer expects and wants to be deceived, whereas the physician has the expectation that the patient will be honest and not deceitful.

It is difficult to prove a patient is malingering. We usually suspect malingering in a patient through indirect evidence such as inconsistencies in history or laboratory data in the context of a possible connection between the medical issues and obvious secondary gain. The problem is with the indirect nature of the evidence which seldom rises to the level of validity sufficient to confront the patient. Remember that "false positives" in this instance can be very hurtful to the patient, and, as physicians, we have a moral obligation to "first, do no harm" (*primum non nocere*). Rarely do we have access to direct evidence of malingering because we are physicians, not detectives. We do not hire a private investigator to film a man playing a vigorous game of basketball who just hours earlier was in his physician's office complaining of low back pain so severe as to keep him in a wheelchair and asking for opiate analgesics and medical documentation to support a workman's compensation claim.

If there is strong evidence supporting a diagnosis of malingering, then the question of treatment arises. Since this is "bad" behavior rather than "sick" behavior, treatment really is not an issue unless there are legitimate co-morbid psychiatric issues complicating or amplifying the malingering behavior that need to be addressed.

FACTITIOUS DISORDERS
Most physicians have heard of Factitious Disorders, and some may even have encountered patients with this uncommon and bizarre presentation. Most physicians confuse the generic term of Factitious Disorder with one of the specific subtypes called Munchausen's Syndrome. As a group, Factitious Disorders are included in this chapter on Somatic Symptom

Disorders because it is somewhat of an outlier and does not fit neatly in any other descriptive or diagnostic category. This is because most patients with Factitious Disorder that you will encounter have clear, objective evidence of pathology that are associated with their somatic symptoms. This makes it unlike other disorders discussed in this chapter that do NOT have clear, objective evidence of physical pathology that is associated with their somatic symptoms. The defining element in this group of disorders is that the patient actively <u>creates</u> or produces the pathology.

A word about definitions may help clarify this. The dictionary definition of the word, "factitious," means something that is artful, contrived, or fabricated in contrast to something that occurs autonomously or naturally. Its etymological roots are in the Latin word, "*faccere*" and the French word, "*faire*," both of which connote making or doing something. Using the word in a medical context connotes a disease or pathological state that is contrived, artful, or produced by the patient.

There are many different sub-types of Factitious Disorders, and this is shown **in <u>Figure 4.1</u>:**

Figure 4.1

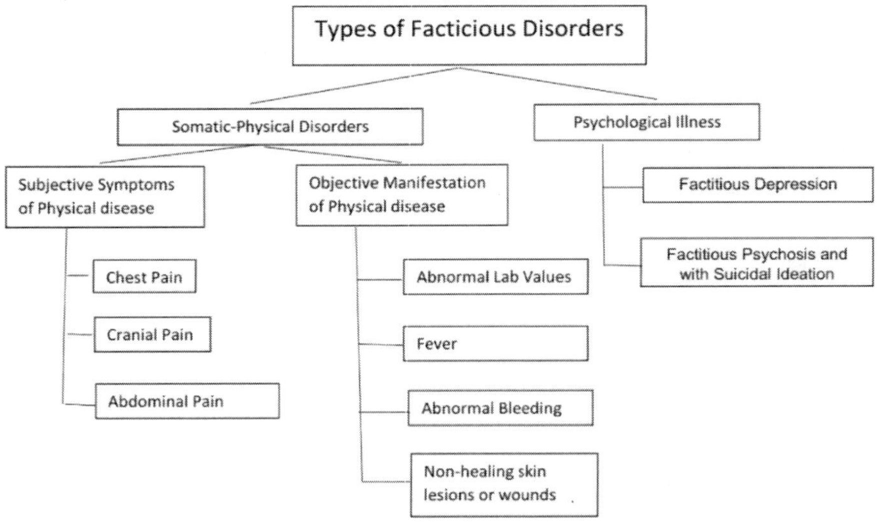

Factitious Disorders can be divided into two main sub-types: those that manifest as psychological symptoms/signs and those presenting as somatic symptoms/signs. It is this second group that we will discuss below. This group, in turn, can be divided further into two subgroups: those that present primarily by subjective symptoms and those presenting with objective somatic signs of pathology. Some examples of subjective and objective factitious disorders are shown below:

Subjective Factitious Disorders:
1. Chest pain mimicking an acute cardiac or respiratory problem.
2. Cranial pain mimicking an acute intracranial event, e.g. SAH.
3. Acute abdominal pain.

With the development of sophisticated imaging techniques, the number of patients presenting with subjective factitious disorders has decreased dramatically. In the decades before CT and MRI scans, it was not uncommon to encounter patients with factitious disorders who bore multiple abdominal, thoracic, and cranial scars where well intentioned surgeons had operated on them based on the best diagnostic techniques available at that time: history, physical exam (both of which are data domains that can be easily manipulated and feigned) and low sensitivity/specificity imaging.

Objective Factitious Disorders:

Abnormal Laboratory values. Examples are abnormal serum electrolytes resulting from intentional misuse of diuretics, hypoglycemia from injecting insulin, or abnormal thyroid function tests by taking too much thyroid medication.
Fever of unknown origin (FUO). This can occur by either thermometer manipulation or injecting oneself with pyrogenic substances.
Abnormal bleeding resulting from self- inflicted trauma (e.g., urethral, rectal, or oral-pharyngeal manipulation) or by ingesting toxic amounts of anti-coagulation medication.
Non-healing ulcers or excoriations of the skin.

This is not an exhaustive list, but it does represent the four major groups of self-inflicted pathology.

In this chapter we will not discuss the topic of <u>factitious psychological</u> symptoms. This is an interesting issue to contemplate, and we really don't know how large (or small) a group this represents because it is so difficult to operationally define and study.

As mentioned above, factitious disorders with physical manifestations constitute a heterogenous group with various subtypes. One subtype is called <u>Munchausen's Syndrome (MS)</u>, and this term is often incorrectly applied to the larger group of Factitious Disorders. One way to understand the relationship between these two entities is to think of a large circle comprising all factitious disorders and to think of MS as a smaller group exemplified as a smaller circle included within the larger circle of Factitious Disorders. All patients with MS are, by definition, included as Factitious Disorders, but not all patients with Factitious Disorders have MS.

This is illustrated by Figure 4.2:

Figure 4.2

Relationship of Munchhausen's Syndrome and Factitious Disorders

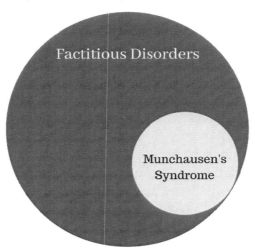

MS is defined by two primary characteristics: 1. Traveling from hospital to hospital, city to city, coast to coast, and continent to continent as a type of traveling "road show" displaying the signs and symptoms of their "disease" to an ever changing audience. 2. portraying their medical illness in the context of a fictitious (not factitious) narrative that is takes the form of a somewhat plausible but very intriguing story. The motivation of this narrative is to captivate and engage the physician and, thus, predispose the physician hearing this story to suspend whatever skepticism they may have because the patient's story is so unusual and fascinating.

The eponym, Munchausen's Syndrome, has an interesting derivation. Baron von Munchausen was a real person who lived in Germany during the 1700s. He was a nobleman and soldier who travelled widely throughout middle and eastern Europe while participating in the numerous military conflicts taking place in Europe during that time. There is some evidence that Baron von Munchausen was the Aide-de-Camp of the leader of the Hessians who fought George Washington in the Battle of Trenton during the American Revolution. When the Baron retired from the military and returned home to his estate in Germany, he became known as a "raconteur" who would entertain his dinner guests with very fanciful tales of his travels and exploits. These stories were compiled and transcribed by one of the Baron's guests, a man named Raspe who later had them published as a book in London where they were very popular. Even today, they are known as very imaginative and entertaining children's stories, and they were made into a movie many years ago. The central facts that the Baron traveled widely and embellished his tales with highly imaginative embellishments is the reason why this syndrome bears his name.

A related clinical disorder is Factitious Disorder by Proxy (or Munchausen's by Proxy). This refers to a clinical situation whereby one person produces in another person (the proxy) a factitious lesion. The other person (the recipient) is usually a vulnerable individual, usually a child, but can be an elderly person or someone who is intellectually or physically handicapped. The most common manifestation of this is the situation where a parent produces a factitious disorder in a child. These situations, when suspected, can be very difficult to prove, but if there is a strong suspicion that there might be a handicapped or vulnerable "proxy" of a Factitious perpetrator, then it should be aggressively pursued. In the case where the proxy is a child, then strong consideration must be given to involving child protective services.

In the case of an adult, adult protective services should be involved. In some jurisdictions the failure, on the part of the physician who suspects a Factitious by Proxy situation, may result in legal consequences.

The process of making the diagnosis of a Factitious Disorder is fraught with all sorts of potential problems that must be carefully considered. Just the suspicion that a patient may have a Factitious Disorder is enough to cause many physicians to morph from being a caring physician to a "detective" who wants to "catch" the perpetrator of a medical fraud or a criminal act. The patient is usually very sensitive to this change in the doctor-patient relationship, and it is often enough to cause the patient to abruptly leave the hospital, usually to the relief of their physicians, but only to take their complex medical deception to another venue.

The other important issue is the "standard of proof" required to make the diagnosis and to confront the patient with the physician's suspicion. In all but a very few cases the evidence to support a diagnosis of Factitious Disorder is indirect, or inferential, and is not based on direct evidence. For example, in a patient with a Fever of Unknown Origin (FUO), who is suspected of self-administering pathogenic substances, a blood culture with polymicrobial flora may be used as "proof" that the fever is factitious. This conclusion is based on indirect evidence.

However, if the patient is surprised by a nurse who actually witnesses the patient self-injecting pathogenic substances, this constitutes direct evidence of a factitious fever. In Law there is a well-established principle that different standards of evidence and proof are required depending on the seriousness of the possible outcome. It is why hearsay (indirect) evidence is not allowed in court. In Medicine, no less than in Law, we should also calibrate the strength of evidence to the potential harm to a patient of being falsely accused of having a Factitious Disorder.

One way out of this diagnostic dilemma is not to get caught up in the process of proving (catching the patient) that the patient has a Factitious Disorder but to, instead, concentrate on allying with the patient to build a relationship that you might be able to continue after the patient is discharged. In this context you might be able to explore the underlying dynamics that might be enabling the suspected factitious disorder. The psychodynamics of Factitious Disorders are complex and beyond the scope of this chapter. In brief, it is thought that patients who develop Factitious Disorders have strong sado-masochistic impulses that usually begin early in life in the context of severe emotional deprivation.

An early experience with a medical event that may have been both painful (physical pain) and pleasurable (caring attention from doctors and nurses). These early experiences may form the emotional context for the future development of a type of "repetition compulsion" for this type of behavior. Many of these patients have an occupational association with medicine (orderlies, nurse's aide, etc.). The <u>sadistic</u> aspect is in deceiving their doctors. This provides them with a feeling of great power over authority figures (doctors, nurses) who are viewed as parental surrogates. The <u>masochistic</u> aspect is the repetition of an early childhood experience where the experience of being a patient and receiving care and attention must be paid for by causing oneself to have a physical disorder.

One last word on the psychodynamics of Factitious Disorders, and that bears on the question of the mental state of the patient right at the time s/he is causing the factitious lesion. There is a controversy about this question. Some think that the behaviors occur unconsciously. Others think this defies common sense, and they think these patients make a conscious decision to engage in these behaviors. This is not an insignificant issue since the majority of physicians are in the latter camp. This causes them to think that these patients are employing the deception willfully, which, in turn, makes them think the patients are "bad" not "sick."

I think a better way to view the mental state at the time of the deception is to view it as a <u>compulsion</u> similar to compulsive gambling, stealing, or other complex compulsive behaviors. I think patients with FD are aware of what they're doing, and they may even have some idea of why they are doing it. They just have great difficulty resisting the compulsion to behave in that way. Some patients with FD have described their self-harm behaviors using descriptions that make one think of complex dissociative states similar to fugue states. The fact is no one can be certain of the mental mechanisms that are operating when these patients simulate disease and illness, but it is probably not so simple as the two versions often put forward: 1. That it is unconscious and therefore not under any degree of conscious control ("sick" behavior), or, 2. That it is a conscious, volitional act intended to deceive ("bad" behavior).

CONVERSION DISORDER

This is a term given to patients who have neurological signs and/or symptoms in the absence of any objective evidence or neuro-pathology that would adequately explain the clinical presentation. The term "conversion" is attached to this group of disorders because of its original psychodynamic explanation, viz., that psychic "energy" derived from unconscious conflicts was "converted" to physical energy in the brain in the form of somatic symptoms or signs.

Regardless of the validity of this meta-psychological explanation, patients with Conversion symptoms and signs are encountered in practice, and their presentations can best be categorized based on the clinical picture as outlined below:

<u>Sensory:</u>

- Hemi-anesthesia with non-anatomical distribution
- "Stocking and Glove" anesthesia
- Conversion blindness

Motor:

- Weakness or paralysis of a limb
- Aphonia or Dysphonia
- Movement Disorders
- Non-Epileptic Seizures

Autonomic

- Psychogenic Vomiting
- Urinary retention or incontinence
- Pseudocyesis (False Pregnancy)

Some defining characteristics of Conversion Disorders are that the clinical presentation usually comes on acutely, and they are not intentionally and voluntarily produced. The patients experience these disorders as having been suddenly afflicted with this neurological condition, and they truly experience themselves as ill and suffering from a disease. Conversion Disorders have always been thought to result from an underlying psychological condition, but the way in which psychological states (emotions and cognitions) are related to the neurological abnormalities is unknown and has remained highly speculative. Nonetheless, we often look for a temporal relationship between a psychological stress and the onset of the neurological syndrome. There is also the speculation that the neurological syndrome in some way serves as a mechanism to provide a psychic escape from the psychological stress that is causing the problem. Recently, a hypothesis has been advanced that proposes to view conversion phenomena as being a complex type of neurological "dissociation" where a specific sensory or motor function becomes "dissociated" from the normal integration and coordination of the brain. In this way conversion phenomena can be viewed as a type of complex dissociative disorder.

Treatment: Studies of patients with Conversion Disorders have shown a high degree of co-morbid mood disorders and a history of emotional, physical, and sexual trauma. Treatment is targeted at the co-morbid mood disorders and, by using psychotherapy to target the effect of trauma on the patient's emotional state. When these patients are encountered in the hospital, there is often pressure to have them transferred to a psychiatric in-patient unit. For various reasons, this type of disposition is usually not helpful and is often strenuously resisted by the patient who finds it difficult to accept that their physical illness is "psychiatric." If the Conversion deficit is primarily a "motor" deficit, these patients often do well by being transferred to an in-patient Physical Medicine Unit where they can have a face saving way of working on the resolution of their motor deficit by gradually re-learning a more normal way of functioning in much the same way that a patient with a CVA with resulting motor deficits gradually recovers motor function through intensive physical rehabilitation. Long term treatment with outpatient psychiatric follow up is crucial however for the lasting resolution of the symptoms and the prevention of recurrence.

In the past, Somatic Symptom Disorders have been fractionated into many different subtypes based largely on descriptive (clinical) and historical groupings. The clinical utility of these classifications is questionable since these groupings do not lead to differences in treatment or to a better understanding of the underlying mechanisms that underlie the clinical phenomenology. Nonetheless, since these terms (or diagnoses) are still in widespread usage, I will briefly describe them below.

SOMATIZATION DISORDER

This grouping describes those patients who have multiple and simultaneous unexplained somatic symptoms that are usually chronic and are often distributed over many different organ systems. These are the patients that House Officers usually describe as having a "positive review of systems." The term "somatization" is used to characterize this group of patients, and this represents an attempt to imply a psychological cause for these somatic symptoms. The term, "somatization," refers to a psychological process (somatizing or somatization) whereby psychological conflicts are unconsciously transformed into a physical sensation. This term grew out of the meta-psychology of the late 19th century (Freud and colleagues) with its emphasis on unconscious processes that would convert psychological phenomena into physical (somatic) phenomena. The obvious problem with this way of understanding these disorders is that it does not lead to a neurophysiological model of how this might work and is, therefore, incapable of being tested empirically and proven right or wrong.

Hypochondriasis: This is one of the more prevalent Somatic Symptom Disorders, but this fact is not appreciated by most psychiatrists since most of these patients do not consult with psychiatrists._It is our colleagues in the medical and surgical specialties who encounter these patients in their practices. The defining characteristic of this disorder is <u>anxiety</u> that is focused on a somatic perception. The anxiety may be generalized, but most often it is focused on the specific somatic symptom. The anxiety is disproportionate in intensity and it is often associated with distorted cognitions having to do with the morbidity and/or lethality associated with the particular somatic sensation. It is important to note that hypochondriasis can be associated with a somatic symptom that does have an objectively defined anatomic or physiologic pathology. In this case, the anxiety is <u>disproportionate</u> to the degree and significance of the pathology involved.

The phenomenon of hypochondriasis (as opposed to the disorder) is quite common in human experience. All of us, at one time or another, have experienced this. Usually this occurs at a time of psychological stress, and it usually passes. Most physicians, when in medical school, often "catch" the diseases they are studying. They may notice a bump or a mole, or experience a strange sensation or pain and attach a meaning or significance to the sensation that generates anxiety. Studies have shown that the vast majority of us experience 1-2 new somatic perceptions per week. These perceptions are "real" in the sense that there may be an anatomic or physiologic basis for them, but they are completely benign, and usually disappear in a few hours or days. As an example, the author, when getting out of bed this morning, noticed some stiffness and pain in his lower back. As I asked myself, "what's this, what's causing this?," I had a binary cognitive path to explore.

One pathway of explanation led to the conclusion that my pain was due to a herniated disc in my lumbo-sacral spine that would soon progress to a significant neuro-muscular deficit that would require extensive spine surgery with a prolonged recovery and an uncertain outcome.

This cognitive pathway would be expected to generate significant anxiety. The alternative cognitive pathway (and the clearly more probable one) would lead me to conclude that I'm an old man who was clipping the hedges the day before and used muscles that had not been used in a while. I would remember that this has happened many times before and the pain usually disappears in a day or two. People who are prone to anxiety and/or who are under stress are much more likely to interpret a "benign" somatic perception as "catastrophic." As mentioned above, the defining characteristic of hypochondriasis is anxiety, but associated with the emotion of anxiety are the cognitive distortions that the root cause of the perception signals "disease" which quickly leads to the strongly held <u>conviction</u> of disease that is extremely difficult to dispel.

This combination of <u>disease conviction</u> and significant <u>anxiety</u> usually result in abnormal health related behaviors. Initially, when these patients consult their physician for their somatic symptom and the conviction that the symptom signals a serious disease, they are reassured when the physician explains to them that the results of the evaluation do not indicate any pathology. But the degree of anxiety is so great that the reassurance quickly fades, the somatic symptom persists, and conviction becomes reinforced. This may lead the patient to "doctor shop," and ask for (and receive) more diagnostic procedures. Their disease conviction and the anxiety generated by this distorted belief soon completely fills the horizon of their existence, and they begin a "quest" to find an answer and a cure. There is a group of patients characterized as "high utilizers of care," and it is largely populated by patients who have hypochondriasis.

Some clinical researchers who have studied this population (Hollender, Phillips) have commented on the similarity between patients with hypochondriasis and those who have Obsessive-Compulsive features. This is an important observation that, if validated, would lead to a specific pharmacologic and psychotherapeutic treatment that usually results in good therapeutic outcomes.

SOMATIC DELUSIONAL DISORDERS (SDD)

This group of disorders is characterized by isolated disease beliefs that are delusional in nature. The somatic delusion appears to be "encapsulated" in the sense that most other psychological functions may not be noticeably impaired once you leave the boundaries of the "capsule." In other words, even though the somatic belief is delusional, other aspects of cognitive or behavioral function often is quite normal. These patients do not have the stigmata of other psychotic disorders, e.g., schizophrenia or Mania. They do not have hallucinations, other types of delusional thinking, blunted affect, or thought form disorders. The definitional boundaries of Somatic Delusional Disorders (SDD) are not bright, shining lines. They are quite "fuzzy" and may appear to overlap with other Somatic Symptom Disorders. A case in point is Hypochondriasis. It was stated above that the hallmark of Hypochondriasis is "disease conviction," so where is the boundary between a "conviction" and a "delusion"? I would argue that disease conviction is often given up (although it may recur) when confronted with evidence that refutes the conviction, whereas this is not the case with a delusion.

There are three common sub-groups of SDD:

- Parasitossis or Morgellon's Syndrome
- Olefactory Reference Syndrome
- Body Dysmorphic Disorder.

Each of these sub-types usually presents initially to a specialist specific to the patient's somatic complaint, i.e., 1) Dermatology (Parasitossis/Morgellon's Syndrome), 2) ENT (Olfactory Reference Syndrome), and 3) Plastic Surgery (Body Dysmorphic Syndrome).

Parasitossis/Morgellon's Syndrome: This somatic delusion involves the tenaciously held belief that one's skin is infested with parasites or other microbes (Parasitossis) or foreign objects such as fibers (Morgellon's

Syndrome). In addition to the belief of infestation, these patients may also describe somatic perceptions such as crawling, burning, and biting which reinforce their belief. These patients most often present to Dermatologists. They usually sit in the waiting room as far away from others in an altruistic attempt to "quarantine" themselves so others will not be affected by their problem. Some will also bring with them small containers of the material that they are convinced are the bodies of the dead parasites or the fibers that are invading their skin. They will show this material to the Dermatologist as proof of their belief. When this material is examined under a microscope, it is usually just exfoliated, dry skin that has been scratched off by the patient.

Olfactory Reference Syndrome (ORS): Patients with this form of somatic delusion are convinced that they have a horribly offensive odor emanating from their body, usually their mouth. Americans and Western Europeans are acutely conscious of how their body smells, and they go to considerable lengths and expense to be sure that their body does not give off an odor that is offensive. Anyone who has traveled extensively in third world countries can attest to the fact that this appears to be predominately a Western phenomenon. Another indication of this cultural obsession with body and mouth odor is found in any supermarket or drug store where shelfs are full of products to disguise odors. Patients with ORS are convinced that they have an offensive body odor, and they can smell it. They cannot be easily reassured when told that they do not, in fact, have any offensive odor about them. The patients are not reassured by this because they think the doctor does not want to hurt their feelings by truthfully telling them that they smell bad. For altruistic reasons these patients isolate themselves from the general public, their friends, and even their families in an attempt to "protect" them from what they believe to be their offensive odor.

Body Dysmorphic Disorder (BDD). Patients with this disorder are convinced that some aspect of their physical appearance is grossly disfigured to the extent that they experience significant personal embarrassment and shame. This disorder occupies a place on a continuum from normal to abnormal. There is a high cultural value, in many Western societies, on physical appearance. This is reflected in the media, in the large amounts of money spent on beauty products, and in the huge demand for cosmetic surgery. This is, unfortunately, the norm in our society. There are some individuals, however, whose preoccupation with defects in their physical appearance is so grossly exaggerated that it falls outside the limits of these cultural norms. These are obviously subjective judgements; however, patients with BDD are concerned about aspects of their appearance that are not obvious to others, or, if they are apparent to others, do not merit the extent to which their preoccupation leads them. The degree to which the perceived deficit in appearance is not validated by others and the degree to which this preoccupation interferes with normal functioning distinguishes patients with BDD from those with more culturally sanctioned concerns about their bodily appearance.

The treatment of Somatic Delusional Disorders is quite challenging and often disappointing. There is little empirically derived evidence that supports one approach to treatment over another. Pharmacologic treatment is often guided by aspects of the overall clinical picture that seem to dominate the clinical presentation. If the delusional elements seem to dominate the clinical picture, then antipsychotic medications are often tried with some limited success. The use of Pimozide (a dopamine antagonist) is often associated with the Somatic Delusional Syndromes due to an old, uncontrolled small series of patients who had some limited success with the use of Pimozide. Other investigators have focused on the similarities between these patients and those with obsessive-compulsive disorders, and this has led to the use of SSRIs to treat these patients. Psychotherapeutic approaches have favored the use of CBT with these patients.

Complex Somatization Disorders: This term denotes a hybrid group of disorders in which medically unexplained somatic symptoms play a dominant role. These are not listed in any "official" diagnostic nomenclature, but many of these disorders are reflected in common clinical parlance among physicians and in the medical literature. Many of the disorders in this category may have some degree of organic pathology that can be detected by medical testing, but they all have some degree of significant psychological amplification. The disorders in this group have two salient distinguishing characteristic: 1. They are significantly driven and amplified by the popular media (internet chat rooms, websites, tv talk shows), and, 2. A strong feeling of victimization and entitlement on the part of these patients who feel they are misunderstood and dismissed by most physicians who communicate to these patients that their symptoms are not "real" and are "psychological" since there is little or no evidence of physical pathology that explains the clinical presentation.

This sense of being misunderstood by the "mainstream" medical establishment has led to self-help groups and advocacy groups that have been successful in promoting the importance of these disorders in the public and political consciousness. Unfortunately, in our litigious society, class action lawsuits have tried to recruit many of these patients to join in legal action against hospitals, doctors, and other organizations. All of these factors tend to reinforce the legitimacy of a "community of sufferers" who see themselves as being excluded inappropriately from mainstream medicine. Many of these disorders are like comets in the sky. They make a bright and shining entrance into the medical culture. They gain a lot of attention in the media, and even in the medical media, only to fade and disappear after a few decades. Two prime examples of this media driven cultural phenomena are Silicone Breast Implant Disorder and Chronic Fatigue Syndrome. Both these disorders received a great deal of media attention and, in the case of Silicone Breast Implant Disorder, high profile class action product liability lawsuits. This was reflected in the large number of patients who presented to doctors' offices having been self-diagnosed, or diagnosed by physicians, as having these disorders. Then, like a comet, their popularity burns out and they disappear from the medical landscape, only to be replaced by a more "popular" diagnosis.

A partial listing of some of these disorders was described earlier in this chapter, and they were grouped into the organ system involved which usually guides which medical specialty is consulted by these patients. Keep in mind what was said earlier in this chapter about the fundamental nature of these disorders, and that is that there is a great deal of controversy over the issue of whether these disorders have an organic basis or whether they are primarily "psychological." Many of the patients who have these disorders (or claim to have them) want the legitimacy of having a truly physical disorder, whereas most physicians and clinical investigators who have studied these disorders doubt that there is clear evidence of physical pathology that explains the symptoms associated with these disorders.

Another way to view these disorders is along a continuum. At one end of the continuum are disorders that have some degree of objective evidence of organic pathology albeit with significant psychological amplification. An example of this is Interstitial Cystitis. In this condition, there is endoscopic evidence of inflammation (and occasionally signs of punctate hemorrhage) in the bladder mucosae. At the other end of the continuum are those that very little or no evidence of organic pathology. An example of this type of disorder is Multiple Chemical Sensitivity Disorder or Sick Building Syndrome. These patients state they are highly symptomatic and disabled by the "toxic" chemicals they inhale, but there is no objective, scientific evidence of toxins.

PSYCHOGENIC PAIN SYNDROME

This disorder is the most problematic of all those disorders discussed in this chapter for three reasons:

1. Pain is, by its very nature, subjective. We cannot see it; we cannot x-ray it; we do not have a blood test to determine if it exists in objective reality.
2. In all human experience, there is nothing that causes more suffering and disability than pain. As physicians, our primary ethical obligation is to relieve the suffering of our patients.
3. The treatment of severe pain by opiate analgesics raises the specter of addiction, diversion, and death by overdose.

Any primary care physician will tell you that they routinely see large numbers of patients with various types of pain that cannot be adequately understood or explained by objective evidence of associated physical pathology. If the physician cannot see any objective evidence of pathology sufficient to explain the patient's pain, they invariable conclude that the pain is not "physical" but "mental" and therefore not quite legitimate. This is particularly the case if the patient's complaint of pain becomes the basis for compensation or disability status with the attendant emotional, social, and financial benefits that accrue from being "disabled" in our society.

Pain that is not explained by objective testing is a highly prevalent disorder, and because it creates so much suffering in patients and its treatment is so fraught with problems (addiction, diversion, and overdosing), it is the most challenging of all the Somatic Symptom Disorders. The particular clinical manifestations of pain are often specialty-specific: Fibromyalgia (Rheumatology), "Benign Belly Pain" or "Functional Abdominal Pain" (Pediatrics and Gastroenterology), Low Back Pain (Orthopedics and Neurosurgery), Pelvic Pain (Gyn). In spite of these challenges, chronic, non-malignant pain syndromes may hold the answer to the neurophysiological mechanisms that underlie all the Somatic Symptom Disorders, and we will discuss this in the section below.

Mechanisms: A fundamental conceptual problem has bedeviled the construct of so called "Psychogenic" somatic symptoms. This conceptual problem is a reflection of a larger philosophical problem that has challenged philosophers for centuries, and that is the "Mind-Body" problem. As mentioned above, when a patient consults a physician for a "symptom," the physician attempts to diagnose the disease or condition that is causing the symptom. The presumption is that there is a pathological process somewhere in the body that is causing the subjective distress experienced by the patient. This involves assaying biological tissues (blood or solid tissue), medical imaging, physiological tests, and a physical examination. If none of these four approaches reveals objective evidence of pathology, the physician concludes that the source of the patient's distress is not physical, it is psychological.
This reasoning has been accepted by generations of physicians, and it has led to psychiatrists attempting to develop psychological theories and constructs to explain how certain psychological phenomena can cause the brain (the patient) to experience a physical sensation. It is at this point that thinkers come face-to-face with a philosophical conundrum that has puzzled thinkers for centuries and that is mind-

body dualism. Nonetheless, generations of psychiatrists have attempted to construct elaborate theories to explain how this can be done, and they have influenced the thinking of generations of psychiatrists. Some of these theories are quite elaborate (e.g., Freud's theory of Hysteria), but they suffer from two fatal conceptual flaws: 1. The theories cannot be stated in such a way as to prove (or disprove) them using empirical experimentation, and, 2. They have been unable to outline a plausible mechanistic explanation of how a particular thought, or pattern of thinking, can cause certain neurons to depolarize in the sensory cortex of the brain to produce the subjective psychological experience of a somatic symptom.

So how do we explain these somatic symptoms that have no objective evidence of pathology? Recently, a model has been proposed called the "Sensory Sensitization Syndrome," or "Central Sensitization Syndrome." It postulates that in the dorsal column of the spinal cord, where afferent sensory impulses are transmitted to the midbrain and on to the Parietal Cortex, there is a finely tuned balance between "upstream" afferent sensory impulses and "downstream" inhibitory and modulating neural circuits that act as a filter or a "damper" of sensory impulses. These "downstream" inhibitory and modulating systems are the neurophysiological equivalent of a "surge protector" that computers and other complex electronic systems employ. This finely tuned balance between the activity of upstream afferent and downstream inhibitory neural circuits can become unbalanced in certain individuals if there is an intense and prolonged sensory ("upstream") input. This "overrides" the downstream inhibitory system, and once the afferent impulse decreases or ceases, the downstream, inhibitory mechanisms do not reset, and the afferent system becomes hyper-sensitized and continues to transmit low intensity afferent signals that are perceived (falsely) as high intensity sensory signals in the sensory cortex. There are many common pathophysiological conditions that exemplify this model. First and foremost is "phantom limb" phenomena. Only a small number of people who have amputated limbs experience "phantom" sensory phenomena, but those that do experience a variety of sensations that are perceived as coming from portions of their amputated limb. It is hypothesized that, following the intense sensory afferent "surge" associated with the amputation of the distal afferent sensory fibers, the downstream inhibitory systems are unable to be reset at their normal set point, and the result is that normally "sub-threshold" afferent stimuli are perceived as a "supra-threshold" stimulus.

Another common complaint is tinnitus that follows a loud or supra-threshold acoustic stimulus. There has been an epidemic of this type of tinnitus in war veterans who were in close proximity to a loud, concussive explosion. This acoustic trauma (or "surge") has impaired the ability of the downstream, inhibitory systems to "re-set" and filter out subthreshold stimuli.

There are two very important corollaries to this model. The first is how physicians think and what they do when faced with a patient who states they have "pain" somewhere in their body, e.g. in their low back. The physician searches for "pathology" that is causing their patients pain. And where do they search? They search in that area of the body the patient says hurts, viz., lower back. But very often a physical exam and medical imaging and physiological tests do not disclose any pathology in that area, and the physician erroneously concludes, "there is no pathology." The physician says to herself, "I can't see it or feel it and all my tests are normal; therefor, there is no pathology." But there is pathology; physicians have just been looking in the wrong place for it. The pathology is located in the spinal cord and central nervous system, not in the peripheral nervous system. The pathology is in the dorsal columns of the spinal cord and the mid-brain where the complex physiology that modulates sensory afferent function is regulated. Even though the patient experiences the symptom as originating from the periphery (e.g., the lumbar-sacral spine area), the pathology is proximate or central, and that is why it can't be seen on medical imaging or felt on physical exam.

The second important corollary to this model is how we treat the sensory somatic symptom. The therapeutic targets are the axonal transmission of electrical depolarization and the synapse. In axonal nerve transmission, we can affect the voltage gated ion channels which are the direct biological substrate of nerve transmission. Drugs that affect this process are known clinically as "mood stabilizers" and "anticonvulsants." Examples are Valproic Acid, Carbamazipine, Pregabalin, Lamotragine, and Gabapentin, to name a few. The synaptic targets in the spinal cord and mid-brain are primarily serotonergic and adrenergic, and there are a wide variety of pharmacologic agents that affect these synapses such as SRIs and SNRIs. There is ample empirically derived evidence that supports the analgesic effects of these classes of drugs.

The discussion above focuses just on the effect of certain drugs on the perception of a somatic symptom; however, it is crucial to remember that a somatic perception does not exist in isolation. From the moment we perceive a sensation, a complex process begins in the cerebral cortex that provides a higher cortical, psychological and emotional elaboration of the somatic sensation. We attach to the perception of a somatic signal a cognitive meaning and an emotional valence. All this takes place in the associational areas of the cortex. This complex process is, itself, a therapeutic "target" since various types of psychotherapy have been shown to be very effective in changing some of the maladaptive aspects of these psychological (cognitive and emotional) processes.

Chapter 5: Mood Disorders in the Physically Ill

One of the more frequent reasons for a psychiatric consultation in the general hospital is the request to evaluate a mood disorder like depression or anxiety in someone who is physically ill. On the surface this may seem like a perfectly simple and straightforward request, but in fact, it may be completely the opposite, both diagnostically and therapeutically. Diagnostically, it is difficult to determine whether the mood state we encounter in those who are physically ill is the same as the entity we read about in textbooks and journals and in those patients we see in our ambulatory practice who are not physically ill. This difficulty is also relevant to the decision of whether or not to institute treatment of a particular mood state.

As in everything in life, we rely on <u>context</u> to confer meaning to entities and constructs. This is particularly true with psychological constructs. These constructs, e.g., mood states, do not exist in isolation. They are embedded in a contextual matrix that gives meaning and significance to them, and we rely on our appreciation of the context to understand them. This is especially true of mood states in the context of patients who are physically ill. The meaning of a person's illness and the effect it has on that person's mood state informs how we understand that mood state.

This point may be best illustrated by how we understand the mood state we encounter in two hypothetical persons. One person is painfully saddened and depressed because he has just experienced the death of his spouse. Objectively, on a cross sectional examination, this person might appear <u>clinically depressed</u>. Only when we factor in the <u>context</u> of the person's mood state (i.e., loss and bereavement) do we understand the mood state in a different light. The other hypothetical situation is the person who is seriously ill with many of the somatic symptoms (pain, severe fatigue, and generalized malaise) that often accompany a chronic, debilitating illness. On cross sectional examination of the mood states of both these people, their mood states (depression and anxiety) may appear almost identical. But when the context is factored in, we understand them (and may treat them) quite differently. Throughout the remainder of this chapter we will focus primarily on Depression. Much of what is said in the discussion of depression can be generalized to anxiety, but there are some aspects that are unique to anxiety, and these will be touched on at the end of the chapter.

When we talk about "Depression" we need to be clear what we mean by the word "Depression," because it has different meanings. "Depression" can refer to a transient <u>mood state</u>, a <u>syndrome</u>, or a <u>psychological disorder</u>. This may seem self-evident, but in my experience it is not always clear which of these three meanings is attached to the word, "Depression," when it is used clinically. These are distinctions with practical significances. For instance, if I say, "I'm so <u>depressed</u> because I have to be on call this weekend when I had hoped to go to the Shore with my family," this is unlikely to evoke the response in the listener that I have a clinical disorder and should be started on anti-depressants. <u>mood state.</u> The use of the word, "Depression," in this context is solely to describe a transient <u>mood state</u>. Likewise, if I say that I just attended the funeral service for my recently deceased parent, and I am "depressed," this statement on my part is unlikely to evoke the response from the listener that I have a clinical disorder that requires treatment. Depression in this context means a mood state associated with other signs and symptoms (i.e., a Syndrome). Yet, if we have all the symptoms and signs of a Depressive disorder, as defined in DSM, then perhaps we should consider treatment with antidepressants.

The above discussion is belaboring the point made earlier that in order to completely understand a word it is necessary to understand the full context in which it is being used. The word, "Depression," when used to describe a person who is physically ill, can have multiple meanings, and it can be quite a challenge to the Consultation Psychiatrist to sort out all these issues. These semantic issues have given rise to the term, "Pseudo-Depression in the Medically Ill" or, as my colleague, Dr. Henry Bleier, has more accurately termed, "The Varieties of Depressive Experiences in the Medically Ill" (with apologies to William James). In the discussion below, I shall attempt to delineate these separate conditions that provide the contextual basis to understand what is meant when an ill person may appear to be depressed.

There are a number of different mood states that are seen in patients who are ill, and to the casual observer (including many of our physician colleagues who care for these patients) this may lead to the conclusion that these patients have a <u>clinical</u> depression. A clinical depression is a complex syndrome comprised of symptoms and signs from three psychological domains: <u>emotion</u> (mood state), <u>behavior</u>, and <u>cognition</u>. A deep understanding of what a clinical depression is requires an appreciation and understanding of the psychological phenomena from all three of these domains, in addition to the real life context in which they exist. Where we have trouble is when we take a symptom or sign from one of these three domains, giving it disproportionate weight without fully understanding the psychological data from the other domains. There are 4 other conditions that may <u>appear</u> to be like depression only because they might share one or two characteristics in common with a clinical depression but are really completely separate entities. I call these other disorders, "Pseudo-Depression" because they appear like clinical depression but are not really a pure or clinical depression.

Some of the Pseudo-Depression states:
Sickness Syndrome. All of us, at one time or another, have been sick. We remember clearly the subjective experience of being ill. It is difficult to clearly articulate this subjective state. The word "malaise" is usually used by us to denote this state. When we state that, "I think I'm coming down with something," we all know what that means. It refers to a subjective psychological state that our body does not somehow feel right to us. The objective and behavioral manifestations of illness are very well known. Remember the last time you had a systemic viral syndrome. You ached all over; you were feverish; you were extremely fatigued; you wanted to be left alone so you could take your misery to bed and try to sleep.

Someone who did not know the facts and observed you might conclude that you were depressed because you were <u>behaving or appearing</u> exactly the way a depressed person behaves. You might appear listless,

less energetic, with signs of psychomotor retardation. but you were not depressed; you were sick, but you looked depressed. Appearing depressed when you are very ill is a normal part of the Sickness Syndrome. Countless times I have been asked to see a physically ill patient in the hospital who was described as being "depressed" when they were not depressed, only very ill. A possible explanation for this phenomenon is that most physicians who request consultations (particularly in academic medical centers) are young healthy men and women who, fortunately for them, have had limited personal experience with being ill and just forget what it is like to be very ill as their patients often are.

The physiological and biochemical processes in the brain associated with systemic illnesses is an active field of investigation in medicine. The details of these findings are fascinating but are beyond the scope of this Handbook. Suffice it to say that pro-inflammatory cytokines and other CNS active proteins associated with inflammatory states are involved. These compounds are known to cross the blood-brain barrier and affect neurotransmitter activity in the brain, and it is thought that this is probably the biological substrate for the Sickness Syndrome. Patients with the Sickness Syndrome are so very common in the hospital, and we are often called to see these patients because they appear depressed. It is crucial that you not assume that because they appear depressed that they actually are depressed, i.e., that they have a DSM-V clinical depression. They're just sick.

Demoralization. This is an important psychological construct which has been described most clearly by Philip Slavney who is a consultation psychiatrist at Johns Hopkins Hospital. (Slavney PR: Diagnosing Demoralization in Consultation Psychiatry. Psychosomatics 1999; 40:325-329). Like most psychological constructs, it has three dimensions: cognitive, emotional, and behavioral. One of these dimensions may dominate the phenomenological aspects of the construct. In the case of "Demoralization," it is the cognitive dimension that contributes most of the meaning to this psychological state, and this focuses on thoughts of hopelessness and helplessness about one's medical condition and the sense that time is fast running out with little or nothing that can be done to forestall an unacceptable outcome. Associated with this central assumption (i.e. that things are bad and are not likely to get better) is a mood state of sadness or depression, or in some cases a state of apathy. The behavioral component is usually one of psychomotor retardation or overwhelming passivity. There is an overarching sense of "what's the use." It is this state of Demoralization that is most often confused with a clinical depression, and it's easy to see why this is so. The two states have significant areas of overlap.

The distinguishing feature that separates the two is the affective and emotional reaction to new information that constitutes the central feature of Demoralization, and that is the assumption that one's situation is hopeless and there is nothing that anyone can do to change this hopeless state of affairs. An example of this is often encountered with patients who are told by their physician that they have an incurable illness and are terminally ill. They are told that there is a remote possibility, though, that their disease might respond to an experimental genetically engineered therapy. In the week following this news of being incurably ill (while they are waiting to see if they are candidates for the experimental therapy) they may appear to be profoundly demoralized with significant features of sad and apathetic

mood and marked psychomotor retardation. The physicians and nurses caring for them may be convinced that they are clinically depressed, and they request a consultation to see what antidepressant treatment might be helpful. When they receive the news that they are an excellent candidate for the new gene therapy which will start the next day, their mood immediately lifts; they become more active and engaged. It is the immediacy of response to new and positive information that differentiates Demoralization from a clinical Depression.

Apathy-Indifference Syndrome (AIS): This is essentially a neuro-psychiatric syndrome whose mood and behavioral features often lead to a misdiagnosis with Depression. The cardinal clinical features of this syndrome are an apathetic affect and mood and what appears to be an indifference to external stimuli. Patients with this problem appear to have an impairment in initiative and motivation. They have observed deficits in initiating multi-step tasks or goal directed activities. An example of this type of behavior is a person whose normal daily routine might begin with washing, shaving and brushing their teeth. If this person has the AIS, they might not initiate these behaviors spontaneously unless specifically reminded to do it; then they will do it, but perhaps not all three of the behaviors. Their emotional state is characterized by apathy and indifference to things, situations, or people that normally they would attend to, react to, and respond to. It's as if they are "disconnected" from the world. Their affect is significantly constricted. Because they may appear to be "depressed" they are often treated as though they are depressed. One such patient with A/I Syndrome was asked if he were depressed, and he answered that he was not; he stated that he felt no emotion, and he often wished he were sad or depressed because at least he could experience something. Characterized in this fashion this state is similar to the "negative" symptoms of Schizophrenia in the sense that there is an "absence" of normal emotion, affect, motivation, and initiative.

As mentioned above, the AIS is a neuro-psychiatric disorder in the sense that pathological processes that affect the Frontal Cortex, the Striatum, and the Thalamus may be reflected clinically in the A/I Syndrome. There is a burgeoning literature that describes the clinical manifestations, the anatomy, the pathophysiology, and the treatment of this disorder. To over simplify a rather complicated process, it is the Frontal Cortical-Striatal-Thalamic Circuit that seems to be the primary neuroanatomical substrate of the AIS. Therefor any pathological process that affects these anatomical regions or neuro-circuitry may express themselves clinically with components of the AIS. For example, patients with Frontal Lobe injury, particularly to the medial frontal lobe, may exhibit the AIS. Patients with more diffuse cortical damage, e.g., Alzheimer's Disease, may have components of apathy, indifference, and decreased motivation as a part of the larger clinical expression of Alzheimer's Disease. Likewise, patients with sub-cortical disease, e.g., Parkinson's Disease, may have elements of Apathy and Indifference. Patients with thalamic lesions, such as thalamic strokes, may show these symptoms and signs. The important thing to remember is that the clinical presentation of the AIS can mimic, in so many respects, a clinical depression. This is a clinical distinction with a relevant difference, since the AIS has a very specific and effective pharmacological approach which we discuss later in the chapter under Treatment. The following clinical vignette illustrates this.

The Consult Service was asked by the Neuro-Surgery Service to see a patient for "Depression." The resident stated that the patient spent most of his day just staring out the window and not responding "normally" to his family or friends when they would visit. The patient was a college undergraduate majoring in electrical engineering and, according to his roommates, was a "brilliant" student. The patient had been at a Track and Field event when he was injured in an unusual accident. A participant at the Track Meet was practicing the Hammer Throw when he accidentally released the grip on the Hammer too soon and it came sailing through the air hitting the patient right in his forehead causing a skull fracture and severe contusion of both frontal lobes. When the patient was seen in the hospital he had a constricted affect, psycho-motor retardation, and impoverished speech. While we were examining the patient, some of his roommates came to visit him to bring him his homework so he could keep up with his courses. The roommates said he was able to do all the mathematical calculations as quickly and correctly as he had always done. His sister who was one year younger than the patient and a student at another college was also visiting the patient. She followed us out of the room and said to us, "That is not my brother in that room. I mean I know he is my brother and I recognize him as my brother, but it is not the brother I have known all my life. He has lost his 'spark,' the thing that is most uniquely him." He is like a "zombie." After a course of methylphenidate over a six-month period, the patient recovered his "spark." He was never "depressed." He only looked depressed.

There are numerous medical disorders that cause or are associated with mood disorders. We will briefly discuss some of these disorders in this section, but it is not meant to be an inclusive list of all known disorders, only those most commonly seen.

Adrenal Gland Disorders: Patients with an excess (either endogenous or exogenous) of glucocorticoids can have mood symptoms that are associated with signs of adrenal dysfunction. These changes may present as either depression or an abnormally elevated mood state (Hypomania or Mania). Patients with Cushing's Syndrome may have prominent features of hypomania or frank mania. Patients with a deficiency of glucocorticoids (Addison's Disease) may appear depressed. These patients usually experience profound fatigue and psychomotor retardation, and these features may lead one to suspect that these patients are depressed. The mechanisms by which abnormal glucocorticoid levels are associated with abnormal mood changes is quite interesting. It is a well-established fact that there are numerous regions of the brain that have a high density of glucocorticoid receptors, so there is clearly a neuro-anatomical and physiological substrate for these changes.

Thyroid Disorders: Either an excess or deficiency of circulating thyroid hormone is often associated with an abnormal mood state. Usually one sees anxiety and panic symptoms with hyperthyroidism and depression with hypothyroidism. This is particularly the case with extreme hypothyroidism or Myxedema. As discussed above, however, one needs to be clear whether what we are seeing is a patient with a depressed (sad) mood or a person with significant psychomotor retardation that might cause a person to *appear* depressed (pseudo-depression) as opposed to being truly depressed.

Retroperitoneal Tumors: For decades it has been a part of inherited clinical wisdom among gastroenterologists that mood disorders (depression and anxiety/panic) may be the symptomatic expression of clinically occult pancreatic cancer and other retroperitoneal tumors. It is hard to know how valid this observation is, and, if there truly is a co-occurrence of mood disorders with retroperitoneal pathology, whether the mood symptoms are non-specific sequelae of chronic GI symptoms, or whether the retroperitoneal tumors have a specific role in the causation of the mood states. One speculation with some partial empirical support points to the fact that these tumors may secrete a CNS active polypeptide (cholecystokinin) which is known to have CNS effects.

Porphyrias: Acute Intermittent Porphyria is known to produce a wide range of CNS effects from psychosis (Example:. King George III of England who was thought to have Porphyria) to mood symptoms.

Pheochromocytoma: All medical students remember learning about Pheochromocytomas that affect both the G.I. and G.U. systems. These tumors secrete large amounts of epinephrine and nor-epinephrine. These elevated levels of biogenic amines have multiple systemic effects, one of which is the production of a state of CNS arousal, anxiety, and panic. These tumors are quite rare, but they should at least be considered as the cause of any intense, episodic anxiety or panic, particularly since there is a potential definitive treatment available.

As mentioned above, this is only a partial list of medical conditions that either cause or are associated with significant mood states. It is interesting, however, to reflect on exactly how these medical conditions are associated with these mood states or disorders. It goes right to the heart of the question of the pathophysiological processes that underlie all depressions whether they be endogenous depressions that arise in people who do not have concurrent medical disorders or in people who do have these medical disorders. Is it the same depression? Or are the depressions somehow different? Are there just many types of depressions just as there are different types of Anemia and Hypertension? To take the example of Anemia, we know that there are different causes of Anemia, different clinic-pathological expressions of Anemia, and different treatments; however, the one thing that all anemias share is a low hemoglobin. The same can be said of Hypertension. Might Depression be similar? Another way to think about this question is to consider that a clinically significant mood disorder (depression and anxiety) is the final common clinical expression of a complex causal chain with many "links." Each of these "links" constitutes a nodal entry point for other biochemical processes to converge, thus producing a final product (mood state) of varying causal chains that have different beginnings and processes. Another analogy is often used to describe this notion, that of a river with many tributaries. Depending on many factors, each tributary may contribute a unique characteristic or "color" to the final common pathway, thus explaining the many varieties of depression.

TREATMENT

Pharmacologic treatments:

The pharmacologic treatment of mood disorders in patients who are medically ill is far from straightforward, and a number of questions need to be considered in any treatment decision.

1. The most important question is whether antidepressant drugs are as effective in the medically ill as they are in other, non-medically ill patients. We don't know the answer to this very important question since clinical trials that evaluate the clinical effectiveness of antidepressants routinely exclude patients who are medically ill from clinical effectiveness trials. We think antidepressants are effective in this patient population, but we don't know that they are.

2. We often overlook the fact that even in carefully selected (non-medically ill) populations antidepressants are, at best, only about 50% effective.

3. We always need to remember that even when antidepressants work, it takes 4-6 weeks to see a clinical effect, and this time window far exceeds the usual length of time that patients stay in the hospital. This should not deter the clinician from prescribing an antidepressant if it is clearly indicated, but if one is prescribed, it is crucially important that the patient have definite psychiatric follow up in the time window where one would expect to see if the medication is effective or not. Many patients seen by psychiatry consultants while in the hospital and in whom psychiatric medications are started will remain on them for long periods of time because non-psychiatric physicians are afraid to either stop them or make dosage adjustments. This adds to the economic and pharmacologic "burden" on patients, many of whom are already on multiple medications.

4. Those patients who are physically ill may have conditions that significantly affect the basic dimensions of all pharmacology: absorption, distribution, protein binding, hepatic metabolism, and excretion. If there is adequate clinical indication for starting

an antidepressant in a medically ill patient, each of these physiological "compartments" must be systematically reviewed to help weigh the benefit-burden ratio.

5. Antidepressants are usually well tolerated; however, a side effect that may constitute a "nuisance" in a person who is healthy and not ill may become an intolerable "burden" to someone who is ill and already suffering a significant symptom burden.

A word about our medical treatment culture which all too often heavily influences our treatment decisions. From the moment we begin medical training we are influenced by the "medical culture." We "absorb" this culture and its imperatives. As students we see this in our residents and attendings. As residents and junior attendings we see this in our more senior attending role models. We watch very carefully how they think and respond to various situations, and we slowly begin to think and act as they do. One aspect of our medical culture that stands out is its "action orientation." The imperative to act is deeply woven into our medical culture, largely for very good reasons. The prime exemplars of this aspect of our culture are surgeons and intensivists. The mantra is, "don't just stand there, do something!" Other disciplines in medicine may be less action oriented and more reflective, but the "burden of proof" for any clinician is to justify why you should not do something.

From the moment the psychiatric consultant steps onto the ward or ICU, there is a built-in tendency to behave in a culturally syntonic way, i.e., to do something, because that is what our colleagues do, and they expect us to behave similarly. We psychiatric consultants want to be recognized as "effective" by our colleagues, and this is often expressed by prescribing a medication even when the clinical indications for such medications may be equivocal or lacking in evidence of effectiveness. It's much more comfortable for us to walk off the ward after seeing a patient and recommending, "start drug "X" at this dose and frequency, than it is to write on the chart, "No meds indicated-will provide counseling." This may be exactly the correct thing to do; however, it is slightly at odds with our medical culture. An internationally renowned surgeon once mentioned to me when I was an impressionable medical student, "Sometimes it is advisable to follow that well-known maxim: 'don't just do something, stand there'," meaning to observe, watch, and wait. In the paragraphs below, there will be discussions of both pharmacologic and psychotherapeutic treatments of the different "varieties" of mood disorders described above, but as you are weighing the factors involved in treatment decisions, always be aware that the "invisible hand" of the culture is always present and pushing you to do something even when not doing something may be the better course of action.

A last word about prescribing psychopharmacologic agents to hospitalized patients who are ill. If you decide to recommend beginning a medication on a hospitalized patient, you <u>must</u> be prepared to do two things: 1) a day or two after the medication is started, you must return to see the patient to see how s/he is tolerating the medication. 2) You must personally arrange outpatient psychiatric follow up. If you choose to delegate this responsibility to someone else, e.g. a social worker, you must determine if the follow up has been arranged. Do not expect a busy medical or surgical house office or attending to do this. They just won't. I would go so far as to say if you are not prepared to do these two things, then you should not recommend starting the medication. If the patient in question already has an outpatient psychiatrist, then you must call that provider before starting the medication to coordinate the patient's care. You may have seen the patient for a half-hour consultation whereas the patient's outpatient psychiatrist may have been following the patient for months or years. Which one of you probably knows the patient better and is in a better position to diagnose and treat the current condition? The answer is obvious. In mentioning these "must do" conditions, I fully recognize how very difficult it is to accomplish this task on a busy hospital consultation service where time is of the essence. Nonetheless, it must be done.

<u>Sickness Syndrome:</u> There is no evidence that antidepressant or anti-anxiety drugs relieve the general malaise (and mood symptoms) associated with severe medical illness, nor is there any evidence that they do not. This situation is a good example of the saying, "the absence of evidence is not evidence of absence (of an effect)." Cavanaugh (J. Nerv. and Mental Dis.) has written about this clinical dilemma, and she states that the presence of significant <u>low self- esteem</u> and <u>guilt</u> in a medically

ill person with depression is usually indicative of a major depression co-existing with a medical illness, and should weigh heavily in the decision to treat with anti-depressants. Often you (the psychiatric consultant) can make suggestions on how to optimize symptom management, e.g., help with sleep, maximizing analgesic effectiveness, and aggressively treating nausea and other somatic symptoms.

Demoralization: Psychotherapy, utilizing CBT techniques, is the primary treatment modality of Demoralization. Many of the mood symptoms in Demoralization are secondary to cognitions associated with the patient's understanding of their medical condition and, especially, their prognosis. Often these cognitions are based on inaccurate premises or are the result of using faulty logic in deducing conclusions from these premises. You should attempt to explore two elements in their thinking, one, exactly what is the fact basis that informs their premise or assumptions, and, two, are they employing logical processes in proceeding from premise to conclusion. Often flaws in these thought processes can be identified and corrected in a 20-minute psychotherapy "session" at the bedside.

Apathy/Indifference Syndrome: There is empirically derived evidence that supports the use of CNS stimulants (Methylphenidate and Modafinil) in the treatment of this condition. The appropriate dosage ranges have not been well established, so treatment is usually initiated at a low dose, e.g., Methylphenidate 5 mg @8AM and @1PM. This helps the patient participate in routine medical, nursing, and PT activities. Care must be given to avoid dosing after 1-2 PM lest it interfere with the patient's sleep. There are few medical contraindications to the use of Methylphenidate. It has been safely used in pediatric populations with cardiac problems and in the elderly with multiple medical problems. From a purely theoretical point of view, one might be hesitant to use a CNS stimulant in a patient with severe hypertension, but evidence has shown that usual doses of Methylphenidate causes an average elevation of only 5-8 mm HG and an increase of 5 BPM in heart rate. So treatment with methylphenidate is unlikely to contribute to the worsening of any baseline medical problems. The exception to this statement is the use of these medications in patients who are currently suffering from either severe hypertension and/or a cardiac arrhythmia.

<u>Treatment of Mood Disorders Associated with General Medical Conditions:</u> The therapeutic effort in these conditions is to begin or maximize treatment of the underlying medical condition. For instance, if a patient shows signs of a mood disorder in the clinical setting of significant hyperthyroidism or hypothyroidism, treatment of the underlying thyroid pathology is usually followed by improvement in the mood symptoms. The question arises in these situations as to whether treatment with either antidepressants (hypothyroidism) or antidepressants or antianxiety agents (hyperthyroidism) is effective. Once again, there is little or no empirically derived evidence of effectiveness of the use of these agents in these conditions, so it becomes a "clinical call" regarding the decision to initiate treatment. This is particularly the case with antidepressants since it takes 4-6 weeks to see an effect on mood symptoms, and if normalization of thyroid function with aggressive treatment occurs within that 4-6-week time window, any improvement in mood symptoms is probably due to improved thyroid function and not the effect of antidepressant medication.

Chapter 6: Substance Use Disorders

Substance Use Disorders (SUD) are highly prevalent in medical and surgical clinical settings, and they contribute significant comorbidity to medical and surgical illness. The Consultation Psychiatrist often encounters patients who have SUD in all phases of the natural history of SUD, beginning with <u>intoxication</u>, progressing through <u>withdrawal</u>, and, finally and most importantly, the assessment for <u>rehabilitation</u> to support abstinence. In assessing patients for SUD, keep in mind the four main pharmacologic categories of substances that are abused:

- Alcohol/Sedatives (barbiturates, benzodiazepines, muscle relaxants, anticonvulsants).
- Narcotics.
- Stimulants.
- Hallucinogens.

1. Alcohol/Sedatives

<u>Intoxication:</u> The signs of Alcohol/Sedative intoxication are well known. They comprise a clinical "tetrad" of: 1) Ataxia, 2) Nystagmus, 3) Dysarthria, and, 4) Behavioral disinhibition that, with increasing degrees of intoxication, progresses to behavioral (Psycho-Motor) slowing, lethargy, stupor ("passing out"), and coma.

<u>Withdrawal:</u> The "trigger" for alcohol withdrawal is not the complete absence of alcohol but a rapid and significant decrease in blood alcohol concentration. One can experience alcohol withdrawal with small amounts of alcohol still in the blood. The natural history of alcohol withdrawal unfolds in a series of "stages". The "stages" are not discrete stages with a "bright, shining line" that demarcates one stage from another; rather, the stages overlap with each other over time.

<u>Stage I</u>: This stage usually begins around 8-24 hours after stopping the use of alcohol, and it is characterized primarily by Autonomic Nervous System up-regulation (Increased HR, increased RR, elevated BP, sweating, and tremor). There may also be present non-specific GI signs and symptoms such as nausea and vomiting.

<u>Stage II</u>: (24-48 hours). This stage is characterized primarily by changes in perception. A patient may complain of dysesthesias, auditory and visual illusions or hallucinations.

<u>Stage III</u>: (36-72 hours). This is the stage where seizures are observed. The seizures are characterized by generalized, tonic-clonic movements. They can occur even if the patient does not have an underlying seizure disorder (epilepsy).

<u>Stage IV</u>: (60-96 hours). This is the stage of Delirium, and it is this stage that is often referred to as "DTs" (Delirium Tremens). Symptoms of Delirium are often associated with psychotic features, and marked psycho-motor activity characterize this stage of alcohol. If these symptoms and signs are not aggressively treated, it can cause significant co-morbidity and, in rare instances, mortality.

<u>Treatment</u>: Alcohol/Sedative withdrawal states constitute a psychiatric and medical emergency, particularly if the patient is also experiencing comorbid cardiovascular or respiratory decompensation. Benzodiazepine drugs are the treatment of choice. Some experienced practitioners favor the use of short-acting benzodiazepines (Lorazepam or Oxazepam) and others favor long-acting benzodiazepines (Clonazepam or Diazepam). The pharmacologic rationale for the use of these drugs is to up-regulate the GABA System that has been down-regulated by pharmacologic tolerance from chronic alcohol/sedative use. Recently, there is evidence that other neurotransmitter systems are affected in alcohol withdrawal (e.g., Glutamate-NMDA, dopamine, and noradrenergic systems). This has led to the practice of adding other drugs to the treatment of Alcohol Withdrawal if certain symptoms dominate the clinical picture.

Examples of this are Clonidine (ANS changes), Neuroleptics (psychotic symptoms), and barbiturates and propafol to target Glutamate-NMDA systems.

The use of these drugs to treat severe and complicated alcohol withdrawal syndromes is challenging, and there is no standard dosing schedule. The key to the successful treatment is to start with a dose and re-evaluate the patient frequently to see if dosage increases or decreases are merited. There are treatment algorithms that tie signs/symptoms to specific doses and frequency of dosing with benzodiazepines. Whereas these are very popular and are in widespread use, they often provide the consultation psychiatrist with a false sense of security and an excuse to not check on the patient as frequently as needed. Not all patients fit neatly into an algorithm, and this is particularly the case if there are prominent psychotic symptoms or marked psycho-motor retardation, so it's important to beware of the "one size (algorithm) fits all" dilemma.

2. Narcotics

Patients who are dependent (tolerant) and addicted to opiates are often seen on both inpatient and ambulatory clinical settings. The two main categories of these patients are: (1) Those who are addicted to opiates that they obtain illicitly, and, (2) those who become addicted, or become tolerant, to prescribed opioid analgesics. Among this latter group are those who have a chronic pain syndrome or a cancer-related pain syndrome requiring chronic opiate analgesics. Patients who are enrolled in a methadone or Suboxone maintenance program are also included in this group. These patients are quite challenging to treat because one must carefully balance the need to treat legitimate pain with the parallel concern of not making worse the acute or chronic comorbid medical condition that is the reason for their hospitalization. This requires a detailed understanding of the pharmacology of narcotics, especially the stages of intoxication and withdrawal.

A. Intoxication: Narcotic intoxication is seen usually in two clinical scenarios. The first is when a patient has taken narcotics shortly before presenting to an emergency room or for in-patient admission. The second scenario is when you are asked to consult on a patient who has been in the hospital but is requesting more opiates (the "analgesic seeking" patient) than are being prescribed. In diagnosing opiate intoxication, it is important to remember that there are opiate receptors throughout the body and the brain. These are described below:

Eye: the pupils will be meiotic. This can be determined by comparing the pupillary size of the patient to a control (nurse, colleague, visitor) who is in the same field of ambient light as the patient.

CNS: the patient will usually be stuporous (the "droopy" eye-lid sign). In addition, there may be slurred speech or a long speech latency.

GI: Narcotics significantly decrease intestinal motility often producing a "silent" abdomen due to a "narcotized" bowel. This can be quickly determined by listening for bowel sounds with a stethoscope.

B. Narcotic Withdrawal: The signs and symptoms of narcotic withdrawal are the physiologic opposite of intoxication.

Eye: The pupils are dilated, noted particularly in a room with high ambient light. As mentioned above, this can best be determined by having another person be a control so long as the control person is sharing the same ambient light environment. Occasionally there is increased tear production with nasal stuffiness and rhinorrhea.

CNS: There is hyper-arousal and extreme physical discomfort that is usually characterized as a "deep aching" sensation.

GI: There is abdominal cramping with hyper-active bowel sounds and, often, increased frequency of bowel movements.

Skin: Piloerection ("goose bumps") seen usually on the forearms or anterior chest.

ANS: Because of the intense physical discomfort, increased autonomic nervous system activity is noted with elevations in BP, HR, and RR.

Treatment of narcotic withdrawal states is important because the abnormal physiology associated with the withdrawal state can increase the overall co-morbidity of concurrent medical-surgical conditions. This is particularly the case if the patient is unstable hemodynamically or is suffering respiratory decompensation.

The objective of treatment of narcotic withdrawal is to replace the "absent" opiate to a level where the patient is neither toxic nor in physiological withdrawal, then gradually decreasing the dose of replacement opiate until it can be discontinued without significant signs of withdrawal. In doing this, it is important to be clear with yourself and the patient about the criteria for success of this process. The physician's goal (minimal withdrawal signs and symptoms with some discomfort, but no major physiological perturbations) and the goal of the patient (to experience no distress at all and maintain some of the "high" experienced with opiates) may diverge significantly with subsequent detriment to the doctor-patient relationship and, on occasion, high drama with the patient signing out of the hospital AMA. To avoid this, it's important to have a detailed discussion with the patient about what you intend to do, how you are going to do it, why it's important to do it, and, of most importance, what your therapeutic goal is and why it may differ from that of the patient. Even when handled in this way, it is still a very challenging process with an uncertain outcome.

One can replace the "absent" opiate with any opiate, but the choice of which one to use is usually determined by duration of action and mode of administration. Long acting opioids are preferred since there will be fewer "peaks and valleys" of serum concentration of opioidss that have a longer duration of action. Methadone is the narcotic that is most often chosen. Its duration of action is @20 hrs, so it is often given in two divided daily doses on a Q 12 hr. schedule. The objective is to first stabilize the patient on a dose that suppresses withdrawal symptoms/signs but does not cause intoxication. It is hard to estimate how much narcotic will be needed since history of previous daily use is so imperfect and the concentration of street heroin varies considerably. Often a "test dose" of 10 mg of Methadone will be administered, and the patient re-evaluated 2-3 hours later to assess for signs of either intoxication or withdrawal. The next dose of methadone will be adjusted accordingly.

Once the patient is stabilized, then a withdrawal protocol is established with daily decrements of the dose of narcotic until it can be safely stopped. There are two methods to determine the dose of the daily decrement. The first is the "20%" rule where 20% of the daily dose required for stabilization is the daily decrement used. For example: If a patient requires 50 mgs per day to be stabilized, 20% of that would be 10 mgs, so on Day#2 the dose would be decreased to 40mg/day; Day#3, the dose would be 30 mg/day, and so on. For patients who are hemodynamically unstable or are intubated, we will occasionally do a 10% (of the initial stabilizing daily dose) daily decrement since this is physiologically "softer" and is more easily tolerated with those patients who are medically (hemodynamically) unstable.

3. STIMULANTS

Drugs that are CNS stimulants are widely used and abused. Cocaine and methamphetamine use varies according to geography, with cocaine dominating in large urban areas and methamphetamines in more rural areas. In addition, prescribed stimulants (methylphenidate, modafinil, and other CNS stimulants used primarily to treat ADHD) are occasionally abused. Most CNS stimulants act on dopaminergic and nor-adrenergic receptors in the brain, and their clinical pharmacology is an extension of the actions on these receptors.

A. Stimulant Intoxication: Psychiatrists and other physicians working in Emergency Room settings are accustomed to seeing patients with stimulant intoxication. The clinical picture is dominated by a "triad" of signs and symptoms: 1) Euphoria, 2) Decreased appetite, and, 3) Decreased need for sleep. Occasionally there may be signs of a paranoid psychosis. Occasionally there may be a history of almost compulsive involvement in a detailed task (e.g., taking apart and putting back together a clock) that consumes many hours of uninterrupted activity. This is called "punding".

B. Stimulant Withdrawal: The clinical signs of this state are the opposite of intoxication. There is a withdrawal "triad": 1) Intense dysphoria, irritability, and depression, occasionally with suicidal ideation. 2) Hyperphagia secondary to a ravenous appetite. 3) Hypersomnolence.

Treatment: Generally, the physiological signs and symptoms of stimulant withdrawal are not treated since they are self-limiting and do not result in any pathophysiological abnormalities. Occasionally, if the psychological symptoms (irritability and dysphoria) are significant, a short course of benzodiazepines offer some symptomatic relief.

4. HALLUCINOGENS

The clinical pharmacology of hallucinogens is quite complex because many of the commonly used hallucinogens affect a number of different neurotransmitter receptors in the CNS. For that reason, there is no "typical" clinical presentation of intoxication or withdrawal with use of hallucinogens. That said, the most common clinical picture associated with hallucinogen use is that of a psychotic picture often associated with significant psychomotor agitation. The clinical picture associated with withdrawal from acute or chronic hallucinogen use is one of a "dreamy" withdrawn and apathetic state. There is no pharmacologically specific treatment for hallucinogen intoxication, except for symptom guided treatment of motor agitation if the behavior is potentially or actually dangerous. In this situation benzodiazepines and/or neuroleptic drugs are often used. There was a concern voiced in the literature about the potential danger of using neuroleptics to treat intoxication with PCP (phencyclidine). The concern was that the anti-cholinergic effects of some neuroleptics might potentiate the toxic effects of PCP. It is not clear whether this was of theoretical or actual concern.

REHABILITATION: As mentioned at the beginning of this chapter, the natural history of substance use progresses through three stages: 1. Intoxication with acute and chronic use, 2. Withdrawal when the substance is discontinued, and, 3. Abstinence. Most physicians are used to dealing with the clinical states of intoxication and withdrawal because the pathophysiology of both those states are so dramatic and compelling, but once those two states have been adequately treated most physicians feel their job is done. In fact, it is just beginning. The emphasis now turns to prevention of relapse by assessing the patient's potential for involvement in rehabilitation, and this is a key part of the treatment of any person with substance use disorders. The newly abstinent patient must be motivated to become involved in the wide variety of resources available to assist substance abusers in maintaining abstinence.

The issue of motivating a patient to participate in out-patient treatment (rehabilitation) for their substance abuse problem is an enormous clinical challenge, but the time for engaging the patient in treatment will never be more auspicious than when they have just recovered from the medical effects (intoxication, withdrawal) of their substance use that has resulted in their hospitalization, so it is crucial that the consultation psychiatrist take up this challenge before the patient is discharged. At the very heart of this clinical challenge is the psychological defense mechanism of Denial. At the deepest level the substance abuser wants to continue the use of substances, and they experience an intense need to use drugs. At the same time they may have some awareness that their drug use has caused some problems for them, but they want to minimize the extent of these problems in the service of being able to continue their drug using behavior. This is where the defense of denial comes in. Denial enables the drug user to either outright deny the problems caused by their drug use or to significantly minimize the seriousness of these problems in the service of rationalizing to themselves and others their continued use. Related to this is the denial that the drug user has lost control of their drug using behavior. Often patients may say that they know they have a problem, but that they can control it or have the willpower to stop their drug use entirely on their own without any help from others. So, it is important to realize that there are two types of denial encountered at this stage: 1) partial denial, which is characterized by the admission that they have a problem but don't need help in dealing with it, and, 2) total denial, characterized by a refusal to see that they really have a problem and, therefore, need help to overcome it.

The CP must try to break through the denial, and this is much easier said than done, particularly when you may have only one brief meeting with the patient to accomplish it. I have found it helpful in these conversations to avoid characterizing the person as an "alcoholic" or "addict" since these terms have such a pejorative meaning in our society no matter how accurate they may be in describing the patient. I prefer to focus instead on the undeniable problems that the patient's drug use has caused. I develop a clear, simple, and concrete inventory of the biological (medical) sequelae, the psychological, and social consequences of the patient's drug use. I use this inventory as a basis and justification for the need for aggressive treatment of their problem. In my conversations with patients, I specifically use the analogy of comparing their substance use with a cancer. I point out to them that cancer will either seriously impair them or will kill them. I point out that, just as with cancer, their substance use will either kill them or will cause serious harm to them and their families. I go on to say that doctors who treat patients with cancer use the seriousness of cancer to justify extremely aggressive treatment (surgery, chemotherapy, and radiation therapy) to "kill" the cancer. I ask the patient at this point if anyone in their family or any of their friends have had cancer and what their recollections were of their experiences. I then say that we have to be no less aggressive in the treatment of their substance abuse as other doctors would be if the patient had cancer. This type of discussion is nothing more than a transparent attempt to justify the treatment recommendations described below, but it does occasionally succeed in engaging the patient in the seriousness of their problems and the imperative for aggressive treatment.

There is a spectrum of intensity of treatments for substance abusers. At one end of the spectrum is in-patient rehabilitation followed by out-patient treatment. For the majority of patients, in-patient treatment (rehabilitation) is preferable since the first few weeks following treatment for withdrawal (Detox) is the time that most patients are most susceptible to relapse because they still experience strong cravings for substances. When in-patient treatment is recommended, many patients reject it outright with superficially plausible arguments that they need to continue to work or their family needs them, etc. I acknowledge their concern for theirs job, family, etc. but then revert to the cancer analogy and ask if they would reject surgery to remove a cancer just because they have to work or their family "needs" them. For the overwhelming majority of substance abusers, in-patient treatment (rehabilitation) is the treatment with the best clinical outcomes. If for whatever reason (lack of insurance or outright refusal), in-patient treatment is not possible, then you must be prepared to engage the patient in accepting one or more outpatient treatment modalities. These range from daily, intensive outpatient treatment (IOP), to less frequent outpatient counseling, to participation in self-help groups such as AA and NA. Appointments should be made for these treatment modalities before the patient is discharged. Information on meetings of self-help groups (AA and NA) should be provided before the patient is discharged. An extremely important adjunct to treatment is medication. There is a growing base of convincing evidence that the use of various pharmacologic treatments (Methadone, Suboxone, Naltrexone) in conjunction with counselling is far more effective than counseling alone.

Chapter 7: Converstoin and Factitous D/Os, Catatonia, Malingering

The unifying characteristic of this group of disorders is the fact that they are most often encountered in medical and surgical settings and the consultation psychiatrist (CP) will be asked to evaluate and treat them.

Conversion D/O

Conversion D/Os are a narrowly defined group of disorders characterized by objective signs of neurological dysfunction, usually with manifestations of abnormal motor or sensory signs. This is in contrast to the Somatic Symptom D/Os discussed in Chapter 4. The clinical manifestations of Conversion D/Os are "objective" and not "subjective" as is the case with Somatic Symptom D/Os.

An interesting historical point is how certain conversion signs predominate during a particular time period, only to fade away with time and be replaced by other signs of neurological dysfunction. In the beginning of my career, the overwhelming majority of conversion cases were characterized by abnormal motor signs, either bizarre, abnormal gaits, or paresis or paralysis of limbs. In the past decade, it is Non Epileptic Seizures (Psychogenic Seizures) that constitute the majority of cases of Conversion D/Os. We don't know why this is the case, but it is probably due to an increasingly widespread awareness of Seizures as a clinical disorder and the increasing sophistication and availability of sensitive diagnostic techniques, e.g., Epilepsy Monitoring Units.

We don't know what causes Conversion phenomena. In the 20th century, the predominant explanatory model for Conversion D/O was based on Freudian metapsychology. This was a very convenient explanatory model since it seemed to fit with what little we knew about Conversion D/O's. The model went like this: Conversion phenomena begin when the patient experiences a significant psychological stress that is symbolically related a stressful psychological event that occurred in the patient's childhood, usually during the oral or oedipal stages of psychosexual development. This stressful event in childhood was repressed, and the emotion associated with this event was also kept from conscious awareness by utilizing the defense mechanism of repression. The stressful event in adulthood that is associated with the onset of the conversion sign "activates" a cascade of psychological phenomena.

First is "signal" anxiety that is touched off by the symbolic similarity of the recent event with the repressed childhood stress. Second, the "signal" anxiety indicates to the Ego that repression is failing and there is a possibility that the memory and emotion associated with the repressed memory will come to consciousness and destabilize the patient's psychological equilibrium. Signal anxiety, in this model, functions as a sort of "canary in the coal mine" that warns the Ego that its defensive structure is being overwhelmed. Third, the Ego "converts" (hence the term "Conversion") the psychic energy associated with the repressed emotion into a physical phenomenon (a Conversion sign). Fourth, the choice of conversion sign is symbolically determined by its relationship with the initial event. This all fit together very nicely, and that is why the explanatory model was adhered to by generations of psychiatrists. The problem was it was a "good story," but not "good science." There were many patients with conversion signs that just did not fit this model. In addition, the complexity of the model made it impossible to test its construct validity in rigorous, empirical studies.

There are numerous observational studies that show an association between a history of psychologically significant trauma (sexual, physical, and emotional) and conversion phenomena, but NOT in all cases. There is also evidence of comorbidity of mood disorders (particularly Depression) and conversion phenomena, but it is not clear whether the comorbid mood disorders play a causal or a potentiating effect in the complex causal chain of events leading up to conversion phenomena. Recently there is some intriguing evidence that conversion phenomena may represent a type of dissociative phenomena whereby complex motor events are "dissociated" from conscious awareness much like complex fugue states, amnesias, or multiple personalities. But the simple fact of the matter is that we just don't know what causes these fascinating states, and that makes it quite challenging to treat them.

Diagnosis: The diagnosis of Conversion D/O is a diagnosis of <u>exclusion</u>. This means that a thorough neurological diagnostic evaluation has ruled out, with a high degree of certainty, any underlying neuropathological explanation for the patient's neurological presentation. Often our colleagues in neurology expect us to make a diagnosis of Conversion D/O based on <u>inclusion</u> criteria. This cannot be reliably done. In the past, we attempted to do this based on textbook clinical features that were associated with Conversion phenomena such as, past history of psychological trauma, past history of medically unexplained physical symptoms and signs, a lack of congruence between a person's affect and the seriousness of the neurological deficit ("La Belle Indifference"), the presence of "hysterical" personality traits, and the presence of primary and secondary gain associated with the neurological disorder.

Unfortunately, the presence of some or all of these associated clinical signs have very low sensitivity and specificity with a correspondingly low predictive clinical value in determining whether a patient has a conversion disorder. We need to make very certain our neurological colleagues understand that there are no clinically reliable diagnostic criteria that allow us to make a diagnosis of Conversion D/O with any degree of confidence. You might think this point would be evident to all our colleagues who refer these patients to us, but this is not the case. Many times I have seen patients with ambiguous, inconsistent, non-anatomical or non-physiological "aspects" to their clinical presentation who may also have odd or psychological "coloring" to their presentations who were prematurely labeled as "Conversion" and have their neurological workup prematurely terminated. Even when a thorough neurological diagnostic evaluation has been performed and has not revealed objective evidence of neuropathology that would explain the patient's clinical presentation, the best we can do is to offer our colleagues and the patient a "presumptive" diagnosis of Conversion D/O.

Once the neurologists have ruled out neurological disease and we are asked to see the patient, we arrive at a crucial step in the diagnostic and treatment process. The neurologist must first discuss with the patient the results of the diagnostic process and the reasons why we (psychiatric consultants) are being asked to see the patient. This must be done BEFORE we see the patient. There are many reasons why our referring colleagues skip this extremely important step, and it is beyond the scope of this chapter to discuss them, but it is extremely important that they (referring physicians) discuss this with the patient before we walk in to see the patient.

Among the many reasons why this is a good idea, there are two that are paramount:

1. Neurologists, not psychiatrists, are the experts at diagnosing neurological disease. We know that, and most patients are sophisticated enough to know that as well. Patients will not have much confidence in our opinion if we are the ones to inform them that they have no obvious evidence of neurological disease.

2. No matter who gives patients this message, most patients will not want to hear it. They will be confused and sometimes angry because of the implication that if their neurological deficits are not "physical" but "psychological." The patient often takes this to mean that their problems are not real, are "fake," or "imaginary." Many of these patients have built their lives around a disease narrative that implies a physical basis for their clinical complaints. It can be extremely disorienting to them to suddenly have this narrative abruptly removed with another that may be foreign and, possibly, to have negative connotations to them.

When I receive a request from a colleague to see a patient for a suspected Conversion D/O, I insist that they first discuss with the patient two things: 1. That their neurological workup has NOT revealed neurological disease, and, 2. That a psychiatrist will be in to see them because they (psychiatrists) have experience in working with such problems. I insist they have this conversation first and then call me, and I will then gladly go to see the patient and make recommendations.

Treatment: The first step in treatment is to discuss with the patient the issues outlined in the paragraphs above, viz., to provide a different explanatory model to the patient that will form the basis for subsequent treatment recommendations. There is no one "script" that works for all patients, so some creative improvisation is called for. I have found it useful to use analogies that patients may be familiar with from their normal lives. One such is the "automatic pilot" phenomenon that all of us have experienced as part of a normal, dissociative psychological process. It occurs when we are driving and are absorbed in a cognitive process, all the while driving and performing complex motor functions such as making left hand turns against oncoming traffic but with little or no conscious awareness of these acts because we are so totally absorbed in what we are thinking about. This experience is ubiquitous, and there are many others like it that can be used. The patient's conversion phenomena can be seen as analogous to the automatic (out of awareness) behavior seen in ordinary life.

The second step in treatment is to think through the issue of the optimal setting of care for the patient, i.e., inpatient or outpatient care. In almost all cases, by the time we are asked to see a patient with suspected Conversion D/O, the referring service has finished with the patient, and they want the patient either transferred or discharged with appropriate psychiatric follow up. This tendency has received added impetus in recent years with the push to turn over hospital beds as quickly as possible to maximize income.

This problem is complicated by the fact that most psychiatric in-patient units are not comfortable with accepting these patients for a number of reasons. First, psychiatric in-patient units are oriented to the acute, pharmacologic management of patients with severe mood, behavioral, and cognitive (psychosis) symptoms and signs, and there is no specific, targeted pharmacologic treatment of conversion phenomena. Second, most psychiatric in-patient units are medically "phobic," i.e., the unit staff are uncomfortable with medical or neurological phenomena, even though the patient may have been "medically cleared." Third, most psychiatrists do not know how to treat conversion disorders, Fourth, most insurance companies are loathe to approve payment for psychiatric in-patient treatment since these patients don't fit their clinical algorithms, and, Fifth, and most importantly, most patients with conversion signs are extremely uncomfortable with being in a closed, locked unit with psychiatric patients who may be psychotic or demonstrating signs of abnormal and uncontrolled behavior.

I think the best way to approach this problem is on the basis of the patient's clinical presentation. Ask yourself whether the patient's neurological dysfunction interferes significantly with their IADLs or ADLs. For instance, if the patient is unable to walk or is unable to use their hands, then this patient cannot be discharged to home since they can't function in a safe fashion.

The key thing is to focus on_function, not their diagnosis, as the key determinant of their disposition. For patients with significant functional impairment, the most therapeutic setting of care would be an in-patient rehabilitation setting. Physiatrists are the experts in working with patients with motor dysfunction that impairs function. Patients who are still coming to grips with the "paradigm shift" (psychological versus physical) of the cause of their symptoms are usually more comfortable with this setting of care than they would be if they were on a psychiatric unit since the former is more medically oriented. Many in the specialty of Physical Medicine and Rehabilitation are comfortable and quite interested in working with these patients, and patients treated in this setting usually have excellent clinical outcomes.

Patients do need capable psychiatric outpatient follow up. This is more difficult to arrange than it sounds. As mentioned above, most psychiatrists just don't know how to treat these patients. An additional factor is that these patients do not do well in the usual model of outpatient psychiatric care, viz., the 15 min. "med check" every 6-8 weeks. These patients need skilled psychotherapy, and, in these ambulatory care settings, they are usually referred to "therapists" who have a variety of training experiences, none of it medical. They feel even more overwhelmed and impotent in dealing with these patients than psychiatrists. The most effective way to treat these patients is, first, to aggressively target any comorbid psychiatric symptoms that may be playing an "amplifying" role in the overall clinical presentation with appropriate psychopharmacologic agents. However, the most important therapeutic "ingredient" is skillful, sensitive psychotherapy utilizing a variable mix of supportive, CBT, and psychodynamic therapy as needed.

Catatonia

First and foremost, Catatonia is a <u>motor</u> disorder with positive and negative features. The most common clinical presentation is "negative" symptomology (the absence of something that is normally present). Framed in this fashion, Catatonia has much in common with Conversion phenomena. The primary clinical domains affected are speech and motor function. Impairments in speech present as mutism which may be <u>selective</u> (speaking to certain people and not to others) or <u>partial</u> (some spontaneous speech but little or no responsive speech). Abnormalities in motor behavior might include resistance to movement of the extremities by the examiner, lack of eye contact, or catalepsy (maintaining abnormal posture). The overall picture is one of marked psychomotor retardation with little or no spontaneous or responsive speech or movement.

Causes and mechanisms: As with so many psychiatric disorders, we do not know what causes catatonia. Decades ago, it was assumed that catatonia was one of the clinical subgroups of Schizophrenia. Subsequent observational studies showed that catatonia was associated far more often with mood disorders (particularly Bipolar Disorder) than with Schizophrenia. In addition, catatonia was seen with a wide variety of neurological disorders such as severe Frontal Lobe damage and midbrain lesions. Neurology texts referred to these clinical states as Abulia or Akinetic Mutism. Based on these observational studies, it appears that the clinical presentation of catatonia is the final common pathway of lesions or functional disorders in many parts of the brain involving many different neuro-circuits.

One explanatory model posits catatonia as the clinical expression of "up-regulation" of the glutamate (NMDA receptor) system which is the major excitatory system in the CNS. This increased activity, in turn, activates a massive inhibitory response of the central nervous system. This model is supported by the widespread prevalence throughout the animal kingdom of increased CNS arousal resulting in a massive motor inhibitory state which is thought to confer, in dangerous situations, an evolutionary advantage. This is certainly seen often in human behavior when, in situations of danger, a person will "freeze," or animal prey will become immobile in the presence of a predator. It could very well be that we have inherited, in some form, the neuro-circuitry that subserves this behavioral response. This model is also consistent with the observations that drugs (benzodiazepines) that decrease CNS over-activation will often lyse or break a catatonic reaction. This is also consistent with the observation that ECT exerts a therapeutic effect on patients with catatonia, since both ECT and benzodiazepines decrease activity of the NMDA-Glutamate system.

Treatment: Treatment approaches attempt to target the over-activation of the NMDA-Glutamate system. The first step is to use a benzodiazepine, such as Lorazepam 1 mg i.m. and check back in one hour to see if there has been any change in the catatonic symptoms. I urge that you be the one to check on the patient and not leave that up to a house office or nursing staff. You are the one who has seen the baseline status of the patient, and you are the expert in these clinical conditions. If, after one hour, the has been little or no change in the patient's symptoms, then re-challenge with 2 mgs of Lorazepam and check them again in one hour. If there has been a significant change in "releasing" the patient from his catatonia, then place him on a maintenance regimen of Lorazepam 1 mg QID. If there has been little or no response, place him on a maintenance dose of Lorazepam and wait for 24 hours before trying another challenge of parenteral Lorazepam. The major side effect of use of Lorazepam in these situations concerns depression of ventilatory effort, so benzodiazepines should be used very cautiously in situations of borderline respiratory compensation, particularly if the patient is a CO_2 retainer.

If a benzodiazepine trial is not successful, then ECT should be considered, and there is ample evidence that ECT is an effective (and safe) treatment for patients with catatonia. Since ECT is often considered to be a significant and labor intensive clinical intervention with limited availability in general hospital settings, interest has been generated in "second line" drugs that might be considered if Lorazepam fails such as Ketamine and Propafol. These drugs also target the NMDA-Glutamate system, and they have been tried with some success; however, there has not been, as yet, enough clinical data on the efficacy and safety of these drugs to warrant their use on a routine basis.

Malingering: The process of determining if a patient is malingering is tricky and fraught with potential harm to the patient This is because malingering is clearly a diagnosis of exclusion and therefor is dependent on the diligence of the referring physician in ruling out physical causes of the patient's complaints. In addition, it is a diagnosis that is quite pejorative, which means that labeling the patient as a malingerer will

hurt, not help him. Lastly, once you start down the path of confirming or ruling out this diagnosis you run the risk of becoming a detective, not a doctor, who is trying to catch the patient out in what is essentially a lie. Nonetheless, we do need to understand this behavior since we are occasionally asked to evaluate patients who are thought to be "malingerers."

The process of malingering physical illness or disability has two components: 1. The conscious and voluntary production by the patient of a medical narrative that the patient knows is not true. 2. There is the presence of some sort of incentive, or secondary gain, that motivates and rewards this behavior. The secondary gain may be "positive" or "negative." Positive secondary gain is the acquisition of something of value, e.g., money or sympathetic attention the patient hopes to gain by his malingering behavior. Negative secondary gain is the situation whereby a person is malingering in the hopes of avoiding a painful or otherwise unpleasant consequence of some other behavior. An example of negative secondary gain is when a prisoner is malingering that he has a physical illness in the hopes of being transferred to the prison hospital where he will be more comfortable than if he were to return to the general population of the prison.

Malingering can perhaps best be understood by an analogy. Think of a malingerer as a "medical thespian," an actor or actress who acts the role of a sick person even though they are not truly sick. As an actor or actress they may be quite accomplished in acting their "role" so that it may fool the "audience" into truly believing them. As a concrete example of this, think of the famous actor, Sir Laurence Olivier, acting the role of Hamlet. Sir Lawrence does a brilliant job in this role, and even though he may convince the audience that it is Hamlet they are seeing on the stage, Sir Lawrence knows that he is NOT Hamlet; he is Sir Lawrence acting the role of Hamlet. And what is the secondary gain for Sir Lawrence? He will be paid, of course, and he will receive the acclaim that accrues to anyone who practices their craft and profession at the very highest level. So we think of someone who is a malingerer as a medical "thespian,," acting their role as a sick person in the hopes that he can deceive his physicians into believing in the validity of his role as a person who is truly sick.

A consultation psychiatrist cannot prove or disprove the claim of malingering in a patient, although they may be able to state that the clinical picture is <u>consistent with</u> a diagnosis of malingering. In order to do that, however, the consultant needs to be confident of his proof that there is no reasonable evidence of physical pathology to the explain the clinical presentation and that there is clear evidence of secondary gain that might be achieved by the clinical picture. Malingering is often confused with Factitious Disorders which we will discuss in the next Section.

Factitious Disorder (FD)

The fascination that FD holds for psychiatrists is in inverse proportion to its incidence and prevalence. At the outset, it is important to understand the core meaning of the word "Factitious." Many physicians think that "Factitious" is "Fictitious" misspelled. It isn't. The dictionary definition of factitious is something that is <u>artful</u> or <u>made</u> or <u>produced</u> as opposed to something that comes about naturally or autonomously. As noted previously, the etymological roots of the word illustrate this meaning as it comes from the Latin verb, "*faccere*" which means "to do" or "to make." When "factitious" is used in a medical context it means that a particular medical condition is made or produced by the patient as opposed to that condition arising as the result of an autonomous disease process. In the Section above on Malingering, I said that malingerers were medical "thespians." In FDs, the patient is a medical "artisan." There is some phenomenological overlap between FD and Malingering, but their differences far outweigh their similarities, and this will be explicated further below.

Clinical Presentation of FDs: There are two overarching sub-groups of FDs: 1) There are those patients who present with predominantly a subjective picture of a disease state, e.g., an acute cerebral event such as a SAH, a cardiac event, or an acute surgical abdomen. 2) There are those who present with objective signs of a pathological state (see Figures 4.1 and 4.2) Forty years ago, before the advent of sensitive medical imaging such as CAT scans and MRIs, and before the development of serological markers of myocardial injury such as

troponins, physicians made the diagnosis largely on the basis of history and the patient's presentation. If a patient with a FD provided a good enough story of a SAH or an acute abdomen, he might convince a physician that surgery was indicated. These patients would often have the scars of numerous craniotomies or laparotomies. In recent decades since the advent of sophisticated medical imaging and serological markers of disease, I have not encountered a patient with FD presenting with a subjective picture of disease. The usual presentation of FD is someone who presents themselves for care with objective signs of pathology. Most of these patients fall into one of the following four categories: 1) Those with unexplained fevers (FUO) resulting from self-administration of pyrogenic substances, 2) Those with some type of bleeding secondary to self-induced hemorrhage, 3) those with an unexplained but abnormal laboratory value secondary to the self- administration of a substance, and, 4. Those with a non-healing dermatological lesion secondary to scratching or manipulation of the skin (See Figure 4.1).

Patients with FDs are usually admitted to the hospital for further diagnostic workup. As this evaluation proceeds it soon becomes apparent to the patient's physicians that there is not a plausible pathophysiological explanation for the patient's clinical presentation. As this realization dawns on the treating physician it may be combined with observation of abnormal illness behavior on the part of the patient such as drug seeking behavior. This may take the form or escalating demands for analgesics, inconsistent history, or unreasonable demands for additional (and perhaps invasive and painful) diagnostic procedures. It is at the juncture of a diagnostic mystery and abnormal behavior on the part of the patient that the physician raises the possibility of a FD, and that is when you, the psychiatric consultant, are called to help.

Many of the caveats mentioned above in the discussion of Malingering apply equally to FDs. Unless the patient is directly observed creating a factitious lesion (which is extremely rare), it remains a diagnosis of exclusion and is supported only by indirect evidence. Also, by the time you are called to see the patient, the patient's physicians are usually highly suspicious and angry at the patient. The practice of medicine is founded on a premise of mutual trust. The patient trusts that the doctor will do everything possible to help him and not hurt him. The physician trusts that the patient will be honest with him and not try to deceive him. When that trust is seemingly fractured, it produces anger on the part of the medical team. When we get angry, we usually want to punish the perpetrator. This is the overheated setting that you, the consultation psychiatrist, is walking into. They want you to help them "catch" the patient at their deceptive behavior. It is at this juncture that you and the rest of the physicians involved in the care of the FD patient are on a very slippery ethical slope where they have forsaken their role as a physician and have adopted the role of medical detective who wants to solve the "crime" and punish the miscreant. It's tricky to know how to avoid these pitfalls and to maintain a position that enables you to help both the patient and your colleagues.

In just about everything that has been written about FDs, there is mention of two things: 1) there is no empirically tested "script" of how to talk to patients with a suspected FD that will result in a good clinical outcome, and, 2) patients with suspected FD often leave the hospital AMA either shortly before they are "found out" or immediately after being "confronted" with the suspected diagnosis. There is no tried and true way to approach this situation. What I have done in these situations is to meet first with the treatment team and review the data and "evidence" to make sure that I am as convinced as the treatment team is that FD is the most "likely" explanatory model to account for the clinical data. I then ask the senior member of the treatment team to accompany me to see the patient. I "rehearse" with the senior doctor how we're going to discuss this with the patient before entering the patient's room.

The senior doctor starts off by saying something positive and hopeful such as, "I think we have found a way to understand your illness and what's been troubling you, and I'm glad to say it is something that we can help you with. We think you have a disorder called a 'Factitious Disorder' and as hard as this may be to understand, it occurs when a patient "unknowingly" (this is a keyword) produces the signs and symptoms you have. We are NOT saying that you do this knowingly (although this is debatable). It is something you are doing without being fully aware of it, and, therefore, it is difficult to control. It is like a habit."

The doctor can then introduce you as someone who can help the patient change their "habit" or automatic behavior. I cannot say that when this "script" is followed that it uniformly results in a good outcome. I can say, though, that when we have been able to get the patient to agree to get help with their "habit" it has usually been with the use of, or variation on, the script above. The key thing is to build the script around an explanation of the patient's behavior that will enable the patient to "save face" and not be placed in the untenable position of having to "confess" that he has lied to and tried to deceive the treatment team.

The approach outlined above is, however, predicated on assumptions about the psychological mechanisms involved in factitious medical behavior, and there is a great deal of controversy in the literature on this point. There is one point of view that holds that FD is "deceitful behavior" that is fully under the control of the patient. In support of this view is the fact that patients who engage in factitious behavior are quite skillful in the timing and construction of the "factitious edifice," and that it strains common sense to think of behavior that is this complex being out of the conscious control of the patient. This perspective sees very little difference between Malingering and Factitious behavior. The other perspective sees factitious behavior as having more in common with dissociative and compulsive behavior. It is something that the patient has little or no conscious control of in certain circumstances as is the case in certain types of dissociative behavior or complex compulsive behaviors.

The plain fact of the matter is we just don't know exactly what the mental mechanisms are that underlie Factitious behavior. In support of the latter perspective, however, is that it offers an opportunity to intervene therapeutically, and whether that perspective is true or not it at least provides a model on which to base treatment.

There is another very interesting aspect to FDs and that is the primary or secondary gain that motivates such bizarre and destructive behavior. In malingering, the secondary gain is very easy to understand, i.e., money or avoidance of something unpleasant or painful. We may disapprove of the ethics of malingering, but we can understand it, because money is, in varying degrees, important to all of us. The secondary gain involved in FD is infinitely more complex and difficult to understand. The "gain" here is to assume the role of a sick person and to support the legitimacy of that role by causing yourself to be sick or ill. This doesn't involve money or avoiding prison; it involves doing sometimes horrible things to yourself just so you can be a "sick person." There are times when the secondary gain of FDs is quite obvious and easy to understand, and that it when it is in the service getting drugs.

As psychiatrists, we are fascinated with human behavior, and if that behavior is bizarre, then it becomes all the more fascinating to us. FD behavior is fascinating because it is so bizarre and difficult to understand. Very few FD patients have been "captured" into psychotherapeutic treatment, but of those few that have been described in the psychiatric literature, some interesting patterns of behavior can be seen in the childhood of those who go on, as adults, to exhibit factitious behavior. Many patients with FD can vividly remember childhood illness events that were physically traumatic (e.g., urethral catheterization, minor surgical procedures), but these painful medical events were also combined with a feeling of being cared for, nurtured, being loved. These events often occur in the context of significant emotional deprivation and abuse. They associate being "cared for" with being "hurt" by parental authority figures (doctors and nurses). They develop strong but contradictory feelings and urges toward these authority figures; they both hate and love them.

Some patients utilize an unconscious defense mechanism called "identification with the aggressor" to deal with these feelings and urges, and many patients with FD have an occupational association with health care, e.g., nurses, nurses' aides, physicians, and healthcare professionals of various kinds. Another unconscious defense that is employed is sado-masochistic behavior. The masochistic part of this defense is easy to understand since FD patients often do painful and horrible things to their body. The sadistic part is a little more nuanced, but it can be seen in the pleasure these patients take in fooling and deceiving their caregivers. It provides these patients who, in childhood, felt so powerless in the face of powerful authority figures with, in adulthood, a sense of empowerment in deceiving these all-powerful authority figures. This can be best described by something a FD patient said to me after I discussed his diagnosis with him: "well it sure took all you 'brilliant' ivy league doctors a long enough time to finally figure this out when I knew all along what the problem was (severe hypoglycemia secondary to self-administration of high amounts of insulin). It was staring you in the face all along. What dummies you are." This person had wanted to go into Medicine but was never accepted to medical school.

Sometimes a metaphor can capture succinctly the elements of complex phenomena, and this occurred once on rounds with a group of medical students. We had just seen a patient with FD and were discussing the psychodynamics of this behavior. One student said that it sounded to her like these patients were enacting a sado-masochistic "drama" and using their body as the "theatre" and us as the "audience."

Before leaving the topic of FD, it's important to discuss two sub-groups of FD, Munchausen's Syndrome and Munchausen-by-proxy. The term Munchausen's Syndrome (MS) is often used synonymously with FD, and that is incorrect.

Munchausen's Syndrome: (MS). As mentioned in Chapter 4, MS is a sub-group of FDs. **See Figure 4.2.** It's important to reiterate that all patients with MS also have FD, but not all patients with FD have MS. There are two defining characteristics of MS: 1. These patients <u>travel</u> from doctor to doctor, hospital to hospital, city to city and some from continent to continent with their medical "drama," playing to different audiences, 2) Their medical "drama" is embedded in a larger compelling and unusual life narrative, the purpose of which is to engage the physician, get them to feel allied with the patient in some way, and thereby get the physician to suspend their objective skepticism regarding the foundation of the medical drama that is being played out.

Munchausen by Proxy: (MBP)This term is a misnomer of sorts and should be more accurately called Factitious Disorder by proxy since these patients do not always travel nor do they have *pseudologica phantastica*. The defining characteristic is the production of a factitious medical illness by one person onto another. There is the "donor" of the factitious disorder and the "recipient" of the disorder or the "disease." The relationship between the donor and recipient is that the "recipient" is usually a vulnerable individual under the control of the donor. Most often the recipient is a child and the donor is a parent or an adult caretaker. However, there have been reports of mentally challenged adults and vulnerable elderly patients being the recipients of factitious behavior on the part of others. MBP is extremely important to be aware of since, if suspected with good reason and supported by evidence, there is a duty on the part of health care providers to report this behavior to law enforcement officers for a more formal investigation to determine whether the behavior constitutes criminal abuse of another person. At the same time, since the legal consequences of suspected MBP are severe, you have a duty to be sure that the evidence supports the charge, otherwise a "False Positive" may have very negative consequences to the innocent person who is charged. Needless to say, this is a high stakes endeavor and must be approached with extreme caution and due diligence to avoid needlessly harming either party.

The Internet and Factitious Behavior: The Internet is the latest "theatre" that FD patients use to stage their medical drama. As outlined earlier in this chapter, FD is divided into two large groups: those with <u>objective</u> signs of pathology (self-manufactured lesions, abnormal laboratory findings, etc.,) and those with a <u>subjective</u> portrayal of disease. I mentioned earlier that, over the past three decades, those with a subjective form of FD became relatively rare in comparison with those with an objective picture of disease. With the advent of the Internet, it looks as though this trend might be reversed. There have been published case reports of patients who construct elaborate medical narratives (or dramas) that feature themselves or others (proxy) in the lead role. The audience is the world wide web, and it appears that, for these FD patients, the "gain" is the attention they receive and the opportunity to relate to untold numbers of people who get drawn into their drama and relate to it in various way.

Occasionally, it can become a ruse to solicit money in the guise of defraying medical expenses. Some of these people are using the medical narrative as an elaborate scam. But for the patient with FD they are not "acting" a role (malingering); they are "living" the role.

Treatment: This discussion is, sadly, very brief because few patients with FD agree to treatment, and of those who do get involved with treatment, most drop out. There is no specific pharmacologic treatment of FD, although in those cases of FD where there is an associated comorbid psychiatric disorder, that disorder may be amenable to treatment. For pure FD, the treatment is psychotherapy, and it is very difficult going. First, the patient needs to be helped to be completely aware of "dissociated" and "compulsive" behavior patterns. Once that happens, then various types of cognitive and behavior techniques are employed to alter and control the behavior in question. This is simple to say, but very difficult to do.

Chapter 8: Capacity (Competency) Determinations

"The definition of mental competency is elusive. To define it is a compelling quest." (Abernathy, Psychosomatics)

"The search for a single test of competency is a search for the holy grail." (Roth-Am. J. Psychiat.)

One of the most difficult clinical challenges that consultation psychiatrists face is the assessment of the decision-making capacity of a seriously ill patient who refuses urgent or life sustaining treatment. This clinical scenario usually unfolds in a setting of high drama featuring insistent and frustrated healthcare providers, an anxious but confused family, and a patient who may or may not be able to make medical decisions for a variety of reasons. The patient is almost always frightened, perhaps confused, sometimes angry, but almost always the object of considerable concern and anger when s/he refuses to follow her physician's treatment recommendations. The consultation psychiatrist (CP) is invited into this emotionally volatile drama with the expectations of all involved that the CP will insure the outcome that each of the actors wants. The consultation psychiatrist must maneuver delicately, but decisively, to make the appropriate assessment.

As the two quotes above indicate, the issue of determining a patient's capacity is quite challenging. This is supported by a recent study (Psychosomatics 2016: 57:472-479) which shows very low concordance rates of capacity determinations among psychiatrists and between groups of psychiatrists and attorneys. If "experts" have difficulty agreeing on the presence or absence of a particular psychological construct, i.e., Medical Decision-Making Capacity (MDMC), in a specific patient at a given point in time, then this indicates that we are dealing with a very amorphous construct. Before we address the issue of how we specifically assess capacity, there are some general, overarching concepts that need to be clarified.

Terms: In general, everyday clinical work we use the terms capacity and competency interchangeably. There is a point of view that holds that "competency" is a legal term, and that only a court can issue a determination of competency. This point of view holds that "Capacity" is a clinical term and is used only in a clinical context. In this Handbook we will use the term, "capacity" to avoid any possible confusion.

Types of capacity: Before proceeding further, one simple point must be emphasized, and that is that capacity is task specific. A person may have the capacity to perform one task but not another. When you were a teenager and just learning to drive, you might have lacked to capacity to drive, and you might have failed your driver's test because you couldn't parallel park. And yet you probably had a high capacity to do quadratic equations in algebra. Only if a patient is completely comatose can we state that a person is globally incapacitated, i.e., totally unable to perform any task whether it be a cognitive task or a simple or complex motor task. In this frame of reference, a patient at a point in time may have capacity to perform certain tasks and not others.

Psychiatrists are often asked to perform capacity determination on patients in varied settings: 1. Legal: the capacity to stand trial; 2. Legal: determining "testamentary capacity" of a patient, which is the capacity to make a last will and testament.

In a medical setting, there are three types of (task specific) capacity determinations which we will discuss below. They are: 1. Medical Decision Making Capacity (MDMC), 2. Maternal Capacity (MC), and, 3. Discharge or Dispositional Capacity (DC).

Ethics: It is imperative to remember that every capacity consult is performed in an ethical context that is defined as a tension between two very important social values in our society, and these two social values are often in opposition. These two values are autonomy and beneficence. Autonomy refers to that social value that embodies a fundamental human right to determine what will (and will not) happen to our body. Upon reflection, this might be considered as the most fundamental right that we human beings enjoy. It is interesting to note that most of us take this right for granted. Most discussions of fundamental human rights involve those rights that are enumerated and described in the Bill of Rights of our Constitution, but the right to make decisions regarding what happens to our body is nowhere mentioned in the Constitution. When questions concerning this issue are adjudicated, it is most often done in reference to the Fourth Amendment to the Constitution which does not contain language that specifically addresses this right but does so in the "penumbra" of the language in the Fourth Amendment.

Legal legitimacy for the right of autonomy is derived from Case Law where legal action has been brought in cases where there is conflict between autonomy and beneficence. One such case that is often quoted in discussions of the right of autonomy is Schloendorff v. Society of New York Hospital. This case involves a woman who, in 1914, claimed that she had been operated on without her consent. Justice Benjamin Cardozo, who wrote the majority opinion, claimed that "every human being of adult years and *sound mind* (italics mine) has the right to determine what shall be done with his own body; and a surgeon who performs an operation without his patient's consent commits an assault, for which he is liable in damages, except in cases of emergency where the patient is unconscious, and where it is necessary to operate before consent can be obtained."

The opposing ethical value is that of beneficence. This social value states that we, as a society and as a part of the "social contract," care about the health and welfare of the members of our society (although admittedly the force of this social imperative can appear very attenuated at times). Nonetheless, this social value has many operational and institutional expressions in our society. It is expressed in the "Good Samaritan" imperative, i.e., that you should do what you can to help someone in an emergency. Closer to home is the social institutional of Medicine and the ethical bedrock on which it stands which impels us to use our skills to help the sick and injured and to protect people from harm. As physicians, we know how demanding and grueling our profession is, and at times we become so focused on the single-minded purpose (beneficence) in battling disease that we often overlook the fact that the patient has the final say in what will or will not be done to his body.

This is very difficult for most of us (physicians) to appreciate, because we are "brainwashed" and disciplined in our medical culture to develop an almost military focus on the "mission" which is to battle disease and injury....no matter what. As physicians we begin to think that the ethical value of beneficence supersedes all other ethical values. In fact, it is the other way around. The competing social values of autonomy and beneficence are not equal in value in our society. Autonomy trumps Beneficence, and the only exception to this is in those situations where a patient may not have sufficient cognitive capacity to make an autonomous decision concerning his medical treatment. In these situations, beneficence prevails because of the (beneficent) ethical imperative to protect a patient from the harmful consequences of a decision that is the direct result of a <u>flawed</u> cognitive process. It is important to remember that the opposing social values of <u>autonomy</u> and <u>beneficence</u> are not equal, and that the scale is ever so slightly "tilted" in favor of autonomy.

The practical, operational consequence of this statement is that the "burden of proof" is always higher when you are thinking of infringing on a patient's autonomy than when you are infringing on the value of beneficence. This concept is similar to the "burden of proof" in Law where it is harder to prove a person's guilt than their innocence. This is predicated on the notion that it is better to let a guilty person go free than to convict an innocent person.

The corollary to this in MDMC is that in "grey" areas when it is not clinically clear whether a person lacks decision making capacity, it is better to preserve autonomy than to override it. Most capacity determinations are fairly clear, e.g., comatose patient (lacks capacity) or a patient whose cognitive functions are clearly intact (has capacity); however, it is the "grey" areas that cause the most concern among clinicians because of the lack of concordance among experienced clinicians that was discussed in the study at the beginning of this chapter.

The determination of MDMC can be viewed as a clinical process that takes place on a "tightrope" attached to the two horns of an ethical dilemma. Making a decision consistent with one value runs the risk of diminishing the opposing value. We have great potential to help and great potential to harm, and this is why we need to approach these assessments with surgical precision.

<u>Capacity: Dimension or Category:</u> In thinking about the psychological construct of Capacity, it is important to review the distinction between a categorical or a dimensional construct. A categorical construct or entity is <u>binary</u>, either yes or no. It is either completely there or completely not there. A dimensional construct is one in which there may be more or less. Examples of a categorical entity in medicine is pregnancy. You either are or are not pregnant; you are not a "little bit" pregnant. Another example is cancer; you either have cancer or you don't. Cancer biologists may argue this point, however, by stating that at the cellular or molecular level, cancer may be dimensional (e.g., cancer-in-situ).

In medicine, we see more examples of <u>dimensional</u> constructs. Some notable examples are Blood Pressure or Height or Weight. It is only by the establishment of arbitrary "bright shining lines" that we impose on a continuum a line that separates normal from abnormal, or non-pathological from pathological. Decision making capacity is mostly dimensional. It is categorical in those states where a person is in a deep coma, and there is no decision-making capacity present at all. Most of the time, however, decision making capacity is <u>dimensional</u>. A person

may have some decision-making capacity but not as much as we think is desirable given the demand characteristics of a specific clinical. These are the situations described above as "grey" areas. A patient may have some capacity but are also lacking some elements of MDMC.

At this point it is important to ask the question, <u>how much capacity does a patient need</u>to make a particular medical decision? This introduces another important variable to the clinical process and it is called the sliding scale of capacity. This terminology is borrowed directly from the well-known medical construct of the sliding scale of insulin dosage where you compare two separate but related variables: blood sugar and insulin dosage, and you titrate one of the variables (insulin dosage) with the other variable (blood sugar). Applying the sliding scale construct to MDMC, we need to ask ourselves how much capacity does a person need to make a specific decision.

Different medical decisions require differing amounts of capacity. An extreme example that illustrates this point is the amount of capacity a person requires to refuse a sleeping medication in contrast to the amount of capacity required to make a DNR decision in the clinical setting of extremely unstable cardio-respiratory and hemodynamic status. Obviously, one needs more capacity to make a life and death decision than to refuse a sleeping pill, and the reason for this has to do with the probability, irreversibility, and imminence of a fatal outcome regarding each of these two scenarios: refusing a sleeping pill vs. a DNR determination. The application of the sliding scale of capacity can lead to an uncomfortable situation where a patient, at a given point in time, may have sufficient capacity to make some decisions and not others.

Up to this point, we have discussed four important aspects of MDMC that are important to understand before you even examine the patient: 1. Terms, 2. Types of Capacity (medical and non-medical), 3. Ethical issues, and, 4. Dimensional/Categorical aspects and the Sliding Scale of Capacity. These four aspects should be mentally reviewed each time you are walking through the hospital to visit a patient for the purpose of doing a Capacity Determination.

The Clinical Assessment of Medical Decision Making Capacity (MDMC).

Capacity determinations are complicated, and it is useful to have a "roadmap" to guide the process. At the very core of any capacity determination that involves cognition is the assessment of how a person processes information. At the bedside, the clinician needs to "follow the information" to determine how the individual is processing the information. One way to deconstruct this process (and to "follow the information") is to employ the well-known model of cybernetics which conceptualizes this process as: 1. Information <u>in</u>, 2. Information <u>throughput</u>, and, 3. Information <u>out</u>. This oversimplified model has been expanded into the "Four Compartment" model of cognitive capacity as popularized by Applebaum and Grisso:

1. <u>Information In</u>: The provision of relevant information to the patient (Informed Consent).
2. <u>Information Through</u>: (ability to accurately recall and rationally process decision-relevant information).
3. <u>Information Through</u>: (the ability to appreciate the information relative to enduring personal values of the patient).
4. <u>Information Out</u>: The ability to communicate a clear, coherent, and <u>consistent</u> decision.

At the bedside, I have found it helpful to begin my assessment with "<u>Compartment 4</u>": <u>Information Out</u>. I determine whether the patient has the ability to communicate a decision either verbally or nonverbally (by writing, eye blinks, or hand squeezes). If a patient is totally unable to communicate by any means, then the patient lacks the capacity to make a medical decision, and there is no reason to proceed further in the assessment. It is important to realize that Decision Making Capacity is not an abstract construct that is divorced from the external social reality. A person may be able to formulate a decision in his mind, but if he is unable (or unwilling) to communicate that decision to others, then it has no utilitarian validity. The most common clinical example of this

is the patient who is comatose. Another example is the patient who has severe maladaptive personality traits that express themselves as a "willful" failure to cooperate with the exam or express a decision. Faced with this type of situation, the examiner may feel fairly confident that compartments 1, 2, and 3 are quite intact based on observations on how the patient makes other decisions in the hospital (e.g., filling out their menu, requesting pain meds, or making non-medical decisions with friends and family). For a person to have MDMC there has to be an expression of a decision.

After assessing whether a person can (or will) communicate, I evaluate <u>Compartment 1</u>, <u>Information In</u>. In cybernetics, there is an adage that states, "garbage in-garbage out." This adage attests to the fact that systems that process information are highly dependent on the quality of the information that is entered into the system. Ideally, it would be helpful to hear, first hand, exactly what the patient's provider has told the patient regarding the issue at hand (Informed Consent).

Usually this is not feasible, so it's important to talk to the patient's physician and hear from that person what information s/he has provided the patient concerning the issue at hand. Quite a bit has been written about exactly what physicians are required to tell patients when they are obtaining "Informed Consent" for an intervention.

There are four standards that must be met:

1. What is wrong with the patient.
2. How the intended medical intervention is expected to help and the side effects of the proposed intervention. (risk/benefit analysis)
3. The alternatives to the proposed treatment (including no treatment at all) and their risks and benefits.
4. The recommendation(s) of the physician and the reasons for it.

Unfortunately, seldom are all four of these standards met, so it is often left to the consultation psychiatrist to provide the information that is lacking if that person feels qualified to do so.

The third stage in my evaluation of the patient is to assess Compartment Two.

<u>Information Through.</u> There are two sub-compartments here: 1. The ability to remember information accurately and retrieve it, and, 2. The ability to manipulate the information in a rational fashion.

Compartment 2-(1) is affected by any process that affects the ability to remember information or retrieve it, e.g., delirium or dementia. Compartment 2-(2) is affected by psychotic or illogical thought processes, e.g., patients with psychosis.

The fourth and final stage in the assessment process is the evaluation of Compartment 4 (the ability to apply the information provided to the individual's specific life circumstances). I have found that it is extremely difficult to get a full assessment of this aspect of the patient's decision-making process because it involves investing a sufficient amount of time to get to know the patient, her life values, and what may or may not be important to her. In an ideal world, it would be good to invest this time, but pressing time demands usually make this impractical.

Once one has assessed the four "compartments" of information processing, then you need to give your opinion, and this is where you need to apply the "sliding scale" concept described above. In many cases, you may feel that the patient has some but not as much MDMC as you would like to see. But remember you need to give a Yes or a No answer, so applying the sliding scale may help you convert a dimensional assessment into a binary or categorical opinion. If you are uncertain whether a patient has sufficient decision-making capacity to make a certain decision and if the exigencies of time permit, you can determine if there are certain "compartments" that are amenable to treatment or improvement. Examples are providing better information, decreasing anxiety or apathy with fast acting medications, or targeting psychotic symptoms. Occasionally, a patient who might have lacked sufficient decision-making capacity has benefited from psychiatric interventions that have specifically targeted "compartments" to enhance their functioning, thereby converting a patient who, on initial evaluation, might have lacked sufficient decision-making capacity into one who now has sufficient capacity to make his own treatment decisions.

Determining MDMC and communicating your conclusion to the treatment is not the end of the process. If the conclusion is that the patient lacks sufficient MDMC, then someone needs to be the patient's decision maker. Someone will need to sign a consent form (for surgery or an invasive procedure), so the consultation psychiatrist needs to inform the treatment team that they need to procure a Surrogate

Decision Maker (SDM) who can function as the patient's "decider." Most hospital social workers are familiar with this process, and they usually attempt to find a spouse, adult child, sibling, or close friend to serve in this capacity. Once a SDM has been procured, someone on the treatment team needs to instruct the SDM what to do when making treatment decisions for the patient. There are two generally accepted instructions: 1. Substituted Judgement and, 2. Best Judgement. The first of these (substituted judgment) is when the SDM makes a decision that he thinks the patient would make if the patient had sufficient decision-making capacity. In this case, the SDM draws on knowledge about the incapacitated patient, his values, preferences, and (ideally) knowledge of what the patient has previously communicated to the SDM either verbally or in writing about what his treatment philosophy is. The Best Judgement standard occurs when the SDM has no idea what the patient might have wanted in this situation and exercises his (the SDM) "best judgement" regarding what he (the SDM) thinks would be best for the patient.

Once the issues of the capacity assessment and obtaining a SDM have been completed, the consultation psychiatrist is not finished with the case. In cases where the consultant has found the patient to lack decisional capacity, it's important to remember that you're a doctor, and doctors treat pathology when possible. As mentioned above, you should try to determine if there is a factor that is adversely affecting the patient's cognitive process and try to intervene therapeutically to restore cognitive capacity if it is impaired.

One capacity question that is occasionally encountered is whether the patient has the capacity to refuse a diagnostic (e.g., cardiac stress test) or therapeutic (e.g., PT) procedure. This question raises the distinction between the integrity of a cognitive process (MDMC) and behavioral compliance. A person may very well lack the *cognitive* capacity to make this decision, but how is a SDM, or anyone, for that matter, going to force behavioral compliance with a procedure that requires compliant motor behavior, e.g., simple PT exercises or a cardiac stress test, or any other procedure that requires the patient to cooperate with the procedure. In these situations, the cognitive capacity issue is moot.

Dispositional Capacity: This capacity determination arises in the context of a patient who, in the opinion of the treatment team, is ready for discharge, and there is disagreement between the patient's wishes to return home (usually to an unstructured, unsupervised setting) and those of the treatment team and/or the patient's family who feel that it would be clearly unsafe for the patient to return home. As mentioned in the early part of this chapter, capacity is always task specific. In the case of dispositional capacity, there are cognitive and motor components that have to be assessed. The standard that the patient needs to meet is the "basic needs and safety" standard.

There are four "tests" for this standard.

1. Can the patient obtain food, water, and warmth? The patient may have the cognitive capacity to inform you how they would do this, but do they have the motor ability and money to actually accomplish these tasks.
2. Can the patient independently meet their toilet and personal hygiene needs?
3. Can the patient meet their outpatient medical needs, e.g., can they list for you all their medications and the times they take them? If they need to self-inject medications, do they have sufficient visual acuity and manual dexterity to safely administer the injections.
4. Can the patient meet basic safety needs, and do they have the cognitive and motor ability to call a neighbor, family member, or 911 in case of an emergency?

Patients who lack the cognitive ability to make a safe disposition and who lack the motor ability to implement it lack dispositional capacity. As with MDMC, a surrogate decision maker needs to be procured to make decisions for them.

Maternal Capacity: This type of capacity refers to the motor and cognitive ability to care for a vulnerable and dependent newborn. This type of capacity determination is rarely performed but in the past, consultation psychiatrists were occasionally called on to perform these types of capacity evaluations. The basis for this request was concern on the part of obstetric staff (medical, nursing, and social worker) that there are grounds to suspect some impairment on the part of the newborn's mother in her ability to adequately meet the needs of her newborn child. Occasionally this information becomes known to maternity staff during antenatal care or in the immediate postpartum period. Usually this information raised the possibility of significant intellectual handicap or the present of severe psychological dysfunction (e.g., psychosis, substance abuse, severe personality trait disorder, or extreme psychological immaturity).

The basic concern here is whether the patient's psychological dysfunction might impair the newborn's safety and basic life needs. Once again, this is a very "high stakes" ethical quandary. On the one hand, we are understandably extremely concerned that we might place a vulnerable newborn at risk for neglect or accidental injury, and our immediate concern, as physicians and other healthcare professionals, is to protect the newborn from risk of harm. On the other hand, there is a no more compelling and sacred bond as that between a mother who has just carried to term and delivered a baby, and to separate that baby from the arms of her mother is a wrenching and traumatic event.

It has long been my opinion that the "capacity" we are testing in maternal capacity is complex and involves separate elements. One is clear, and that is whether there is present clear evidence of psychopathology that would make it *foreseeable* that it would impair the mother's ability to care for the newborn. But other elements are equally important. One of these elements is social, and the questions that must be answered are whether the mother has previously come to the attention of Child Protective Services for abuse or neglect of a child. We need to be assured that a child of the mother has never been removed from her custody for whatever reason. Related to the social concerns is whether the patient has a safe place to live with water and heat and the necessary finances to buy food, diapers, and clothes for the newborn. It needs to be determined if there is a capable adult living with the patient and her newborn who can support, help, and take over the care of the newborn if that becomes necessary. The third element is whether the patient has the intellectual capability to know when and how to feed the newborn and to know when and how to change its diapers. Another important issue is whether the mother is "bonding" with the newborn. Does she want to hold the baby and rock it when it is distressed, or does she ignore the baby and watch TV seemingly oblivious to the presence of the newborn. This aspect of maternal capacity is best determined by direct observation by the maternity unit nurses who can evaluate each component of this aspect of care. Particular attention must be paid to the presence of any motor impairment (Muscular Dystrophy or Multiple Sclerosis) that, even in the presence of clear cognitive capacity, might impair the ability of the mother to adequately and safely care for her newborn. Viewed in this fashion, Maternal Capacity is a "Tri-Partite" capacity evaluation with Social Work, Nursing, and Psychiatry all contributing information from their area of professional expertise with the patient's obstetrician making the final determination.

AMA Discharges: CPs are often consulted by their colleagues to determine the decision making capacity of their patients who wish to be discharged from inpatient treatment against medical advice. The basic approach to this type of capacity determination is the same as has been outlined above; however, there is an added dimension to the factors that must be calibrated in the "sliding scale," risk/benefit analysis that needs to be emphasized. There is evidence that the large majority of patients who request discharge AMA have comorbid substance abuse problems, and their wish to satisfy their cravings for substances overrides the perceived benefit to continue life sustaining treatment that can only be provided in an inpatient hospital setting.

The patient requesting discharge AMA may be fully cognizant of the benefits of continued treatment in the hospital, and they may be equally aware of the dangers to them of foregoing that treatment. The basic issue here is whether their decision is more heavily weighted in favor of an immediate or short term perceived benefit to them of satisfying the intense hunger or craving for their substance of choice compared to the long-term perceived benefit of improving their health. This is a basic aspect of our human psychology, and we see it operating in many areas of human psychology, e.g., eating a rich dessert (because we crave it) knowing that it may adversely affect our blood sugar and make our diabetes harder to control. When we encounter evidence of this type of behavior in everyday life, we view it negatively, and we characterize it with pejorative adjectives, e.g., "short-sighted," "impulsive," "immature," "reckless," or just plain "stupid." The issue here is whether "stupid" behavior is a sufficient reason to infringe on a patient's autonomy or liberty rights, and, if so, at what point.

A second important issue to consider in determining the decision-making capacity of a patient requesting AMA discharge is to realize that when overruling a patient's request to leave the hospital you are creating a situation of double indemnity. When you treat an incapacitated patient against his will, you are infringing on that patient's psychological autonomy. You are doing something to the integrity of their body that they have denied you the permission to do. In overruling a patient's request to leave the hospital and forego treatment, you are, in effect, adding an additional important ethical layer to the equation. You are not only infringing on their autonomy; you are also infringing on their liberty. You are basically making them a prisoner because you have deprived them of their basic right of liberty. You are imprisoning them in their hospital room and severely limiting their ability to move about. Operationally, this means the "bar" or "threshold" of denying a patient their liberty rights has been raised, and to meet this higher standard there has to be clearer evidence of compromised cognitive functioning in making the determination of decision making incapacity.

In summary, it is important to remember that all Capacity Determinations are task specific, and all capacity determinations are done in an ethical context that takes place in the "tension" between the important competing social values of autonomy and beneficence. As you walk away from having completed each capacity determination you should ask yourself whether you have compromised one social value in favor of the other. The answer will almost always be "yes" (except in clear cases of incapacity, e.g., coma), but you should always question whether you have placed your "finger too strongly on the scale" in favor of one at the expense of the other.

Chapter 9: Assessment of the Organ Transplant Candidate

Transplantation Medicine is a rapidly growing area of medicine and surgery. Associated with this field of medicine are <u>three</u> overarching issues that structure our involvement, as consultation psychiatrists, in the process of evaluating potential transplant candidates (both organ recipients and donors).

<u>Supply and Demand</u>

The <u>demand</u> (need) for organs and tissues for transplantation far outstrips the <u>supply</u> of suitable organs and tissues. This stark fact imposes an unavoidable imperative for transplant teams to determine who is a suitable candidate and who is not. Although we don't like to state it in these terms because of the pejorative social, ethical, and political connotations, this process constitutes rationing of scarce health care resources. This does not mean that the consultation psychiatrist is going to be the "final decider," but it does mean that s/he will provide important clinical input into the final decision of who will or will not receive a potentially life-saving or sustaining surgical procedure. The ethical high stakes nature of this process is the consequence of any final yes/no decision. If it is decided that the candidate we have evaluated is not "suitable," then there is a high likelihood that that patient may die or live out a shortened life of high morbidity and decreased function. If it is decided that the candidate is "suitable" and receives an organ, then that means that there is one fewer organ available for someone else to have, and that "unknown" (to us) patient may die for lack of the organ that went to our candidate.

What this means to the consultation psychiatrist, who is walking through the halls of the hospital on the way to evaluate a candidate's suitability for a transplant, is that this is a very serious process with extremely important consequences, and it demands great care and diligence. It is very tempting and emotionally convenient to approach this clinical evaluation with a type of "tunnel vision" that enables you to see this process as just a simple clinical evaluation of one patient's clinical status. This "tunnel vision" may obscure seeing and appreciating the larger social and ethical context that exists outside the immediate interaction with the patient in front of you.

Organ Transplantation is a "gift"

The receipt of an organ that will save a life or sustain a life is a tremendous gift of an exceedingly rare (and therefore valuable) social resource. We need to be sure that the recipient will "nurture and protect" this gift as diligently as possible, and the specifics of this will be discussed in detail below.

Psychological aspects of donating and receiving the "gift" of an organ.

Giving a part of your body (donor) or receiving a body part from another person (recipient), whom you may or may not know, is not a "neutral" psychological event. Different organs and body parts have vastly different psychological meanings to people. We know that the heart has many symbolic meanings to people. Likewise, in the minds of people unfamiliar with human anatomy and physiology, the kidney is often associated with the genitourinary system, and this association may take on added symbolic meaning as a part of a person's sexual anatomy and function. As different organs and body parts are transplanted (face, penis, uterus, hands) the psychological dimension of transplantation becomes even more important. Organ and tissue recipients who are unfamiliar with the donor often wonder about the gender, race, or religion of the donor, and they wonder whether the incorporation if the transplanted organ changes their own identity. These are just things to keep in mind when you evaluate either a donor or a recipient of an organ or tissue transplant.

The Evaluation Process:

Informed Consent: The Consultation Psychiatrist should first determine the adequacy of the informed consent by asking the patient what s/he understands is involved in the surgery and aftercare. In my experience, rarely do patients have an adequate understanding of the surgery involved and the aftercare involved. There are two reasons for this. First, most physicians do not take the time to do a thorough and detailed description of the surgery and aftercare, and, second, even when they do provide adequate information, many patients remember only a fraction of what they are told. The CP may need to supplement the patient's understanding of what is involved in the surgery, but, of most importance, the significant life style change involved in the post-operative period and the necessity for life-long adherence to taking immunosuppressant drugs and maintaining close contact with medical follow up. The patient needs to have a clear and concrete understanding of what will happen if there is less than optimal adherence to immunosuppressants.

"Stewardship" of the transplant: This is the most important part of the psychiatric evaluation of the transplant candidate, and it incorporates points one and two discussed in the introduction above. The patient has been given a "gift" of an incredibly scarce and valuable social resource: an organ or a tissue. It is our job as consultation psychiatrists to determine the extent to which the patient has the psychological and social resources to insure the care and protection of this extremely valuable "gift." We want to assess whether the patient may be at risk for harming this "adopted" organ, either actively or passively. Although it is thankfully rare, the worst-case scenario of a patient actively harming the "gift" is to commit suicide after surgery. The more likely concern is that the patient will "passively" harm the gifted organ by not caring for it adequately through non-compliance with a complicated medical and pharmacologic regimen. The survivability of a transplanted organ is directly related to the degree of close compliance post-operatively with a rigorous and life-long adherence to taking immunosuppressant medications and follow up with the transplant team.

Compliance with medications and follow up care is difficult to predict, but the best way to predict the future is to look at the past in terms of compliance with <u>medications</u>, <u>diet</u>, and <u>doctor visits</u>. I usually begin by asking the patient if s/he knows what medications they are taking, how frequently they take them, and for what reasons. I ask about dietary compliance and compliance with doctor and clinic visits. The answers to these questions do not equate to good or poor compliance in the post-transplant period, but they do provide some indication. Related to compliance issues are psychological disorders that might be expected to have a negative effect on compliance. Alcohol and substance abuse will have a major effect on the likelihood of compliance. Likewise, severe personality trait disorders, depression, bipolar disorder, and psychosis all can be expected to have a negative effect on compliance with a rigorous postoperative regimen.

Social factors are extremely important to assess. It's hard to imagine a more rigorous and demanding medical-surgical intervention and post-operative course, and potential candidates will need to have adequate and stable social supports. There are a number of structured, clinical assessment scales that have been developed to guide the consultation psychiatrist in performing this evaluation. Most of these scales evaluate the following data domains:

- Social Support.
- Psychological health (psychiatric disorders and neurocognitive functioning, such as executive function and memory function)
- Lifestyle factors (including substance use and compliance with medications).
- Full and complete understanding of the entire transplant process.

<u>Our Recommendation</u>: The final decision on whether the patient will be accepted as a candidate for transplant is not yours to make. It is made by the Transplant Team where data from multiple sources are reviewed and weighed; however, the psycho-social input is given significant weight in the final decision. There is the belief that psychosocial risk factors are associated with poor outcomes. The majority of studies (but

not all) looking at this association has supported the notion that high psychosocial risk factors are associated with poorer outcomes.

One perspective that has obvious merit is to include in the recommendation specific proposals to target deficits in psychological and social functioning to ensure that the patient is at the "top of his game" as they start the transplant process. In other words, we don't want to provide just a psycho-social "snapshot" of how the patient is at a given point in time, but we want to include a plan of action of how to aggressively maximize their psycho-social adjustment. Many post-op transplant patients will need some form of psychiatric follow up to ensure that identified psychosocial deficits are being monitored and maximally treated. In the immediate post-operative phase, it is important to monitor for delirium and the rare but clinically important leukoencephalopathy associated with immunosuppressants. As patients recover from the transplant surgery and begin to adjust to life with their new organ, they may experience some psychological reactions mentioned above. One such reaction is "survivor guilt." The feeling that their new life comes at the expense of someone else's death. Emotional reactions to certain types of non-lifesaving or sustaining transplants, such as face, uterus, limb may raise questions and feelings about altered identity and difficulty in integrating the new body part into their self-image.

Chapter 10: The Patient with Cancer

As consultation psychiatrists, we are often asked to participate in the care of patients who have cancer. This occurs both in the inpatient and outpatient clinical settings. It is perhaps superfluous to say that having cancer is different from having other diseases, no matter how serious, because cancer has a unique psychological, social, and cultural significance that transcends the basic biological realities of what is occurring at the cellular, tissue, and organ level. Susan Sontag, in her book, "Illness as a Metaphor," writes eloquently about the complex emotional issues that become attached to the biological process of disease (and cancer). Cancer means vastly different things to different people, and this depends on that person's unique history (family member with cancer), the socio-cultural meaning of cancer for that person, and the person's psychological history and ways that they have responded to illness events in the past. As you are preparing to meet a patient with cancer, you should remind yourself of these overarching issues.

<u>Evaluation and Treatment:</u> When evaluating any psychiatric patient, it is a conceptual "convenience" to distinguish psychological phenomena as being caused by either <u>psychological</u> or <u>biological</u> etiologies. Clinically, it is very difficult to make this distinction because the two categories often overlap and, at their root cause, all psychological phenomena are ultimately biological in origin. Nonetheless, we will utilize this distinction in the discussion below.

The two primary psychological issues to explore in patients with cancer are <u>anxiety and depression</u> and the mood-specific cognitions that are associated with them. Many cancer patients are terribly sick (physically) either from the cancer biology and its constitutional effects and/or its treatment (surgery, chemotherapy, and radiation). This comorbidity raises some of the issues discussed in Chapter 5 (Mood Disorders), and makes it difficult to know exactly what type of depression and/or anxiety we are dealing with and whether it is the type of mood symptom that responds to medications. One important aspect of a cancer patient's reaction to their illness is the often encountered thought that a lifestyle or other type of behavior may have contributed to the etiology of the cancer. Over the past three decades, the lay media has fostered the belief that bad life choices, stress, poor sleep, too little exercise, and other life issues either cause or predispose people to having cancer. There is little if any good empirically derived scientific evidence to support these beliefs (except, of course, exposure to certain environmental toxins, e.g., tobacco smoke). There is a tremendous negative effect associated with these beliefs because it makes the patient feel responsible, and therefor guilty, for the fact that they have cancer. This guilt is magnified by the feeling that not only are they responsible for their own illness, in some fashion, but are also responsible for the pain and suffering their illness may impose on family and close friends, particularly young children. This set of beliefs literally adds "insult to injury." This belief, if present, must be the target of psychotherapy to help relieve the patient of the terrible emotional burden (physical and psychological) of having cancer.

Patients with severe psychopathology such as psychosis, depression, bipolar disorder, substance abuse, and severe personality trait disorders are, obviously, not "immune" to developing cancer, and their psychiatric symptoms must be treated as aggressively as they would in any other context. However, the risks and burdens these disorders impose on the often rigorous treatment protocols required for successful treatment of their cancer are tremendous, and therefore deserve even more aggressive treatment, frequent follow up, and monitoring of treatment compliance. Patients with these more serious psychiatric disorders are prone to refuse treatment and to be non-compliant with aspects of their treatment. In addition, they may manifest very maladaptive and provocative behaviors towards their caregivers that seriously challenge the doctor-patient relationship.

Patients with cancer mobilize and utilize a large "repertoire" of psychological defenses and coping mechanisms in the service of dealing with the emotions associated with cancer and its treatment. One defense that is often manifest in this context is <u>Denial</u>. Denial can occasionally serve a useful purpose by keeping out of conscious awareness certain facts (e.g., poor prognosis) associated with cancer, and in this way help the patient lead some semblance of a normal life without the constant knowledge that one's life is foreshortened. However, the use of Denial can be extremely maladaptive if it interferes with treatment compliance or it enables a cancer patient to make life plans that are unrealistic, given a particular prognosis, that might have a destructive impact on others (family, friends), e.g., emptying a savings account to pay for a one year, around-the-world cruise when it is clear that the patient's survival will not exceed a few months. The psychological treatment of the cancer patient requires a careful analysis of a patient's repertoire of defenses and coping mechanisms with the goal of supporting and maximizing those defenses that are mature and adaptive (e.g. sublimation, altruism, intellectualization, humor, suppression) and guarding against those defenses that are maladaptive (e.g., repression, acting out, displacement, and denial).

The pharmacologic treatment of psychiatric symptoms in the cancer patient is basically similar to that with any other patient with comorbid psychiatric and medical conditions. The major concern, before initiating psychopharmacologic treatment, is to carefully review the specific pathophysiology of the patient's cancer and the effects of any treatment the patient is receiving to insure there will be no adverse interaction between the pharmacology (absorption, distribution, bioavailability, and metabolism) of the drug you are prescribing and the pathology of the patient's cancer or treatment.

One example of this type of interaction that is often quoted is the potential adverse interaction of paroxetine and tamoxifen, a chemotherapeutic agent used in the treatment of certain breast cancers. Tamoxifen is a "pro-drug" that is not therapeutically active, and it requires metabolism by one of the cytochrome P-450 enzymes to produce a metabolite that has anti-neoplastic action. Paroxetine inhibits the action of this particular enzyme with the result that it may decrease blood levels of the therapeutically active moiety of tamoxifen. Recent studies have questioned whether the decrease in plasma levels of the active metabolite of tamoxifen is actually that significant in patients who are also taking paroxetine; however, the principle is important, and it reminds us that before prescribing medications to patients with cancer, we must be sure we understand the potential interactions of the drug we're prescribing with the cancer pathology and treatment of the patient. These considerations will be discussed in more detail below in Chapter 13, "Psychopharmacology in the Medically Ill Patient."

In both the initial evaluation and the follow up care of the cancer patient, it is important to be aware of the possibility that some or all of the psychiatric clinical presentation may be the clinical expression of a direct or indirect effect of the tumor on brain tissue. The structural and functional integrity of brain tissue function is sensitive to the mass effect of the tumor on brain tissue integrity. This can occur with both primary brain tumors and metastases to the brain from tumors outside the brain. There is also an indirect effect on brain function by certain extra-cerebral tumors via hormonal or immunological mechanisms. A rare but striking example of this category of pathology are paraneoplastic syndromes, particularly those producing an autoimmune encephalitis. This is important to be aware of since the earliest manifestations of these syndromes may be the sudden onset of focal neurological deficits and psychiatric symptoms, such as anxiety, agitation, insomnia, psychotic symptoms, and decreased memory. These neuropsychiatric syndromes can be devastating to patients. Their early recognition can lead to targeted treatment of the immune pathology with possible sparing of months of debilitating symptoms and loss of motor and cognitive function.

There are other tumors that can have distal effects on brain (psychological) function. Pheochromocytomas may first present with sudden onset of extreme anxiety associated with signs of autonomic nervous system abnormalities. These symptom presentations may seem like panic attacks in the sense that they may not be associated with any emotional "triggers." Depending on the anatomical location of the pheochromocytoma (usually in the GI tract or pelvis), the symptoms may be triggered by the function of the organ the tumor is attached to, e.g., GI track (defecation) or Bladder (voiding).

Another interesting example of the "distal" effect of tumors on brain function and symptomatology is the association between certain retroperitoneal tumors (sarcomas) and severe anxiety and depression. This association has been observed and noted in gastroenterology textbooks for decades. It has been difficult to sort out the specific nature of this connection (if, indeed, there is one), but there is a putative mechanism to explain this association, and that is some retroperitoneal tumors are thought to secrete a CNS active polypeptide (e.g., cholecystokinin) which has been shown to be anxiogenic.

Chapter 11: The Dying Patient

"Dying is not a psychiatric disorder"
-John Fryer, MD

The central question that must be addressed in any discussion of psychiatrists being involved in the care of the dying patient is, 'Why?' What role does a psychiatrist play in the care of someone who is dying? This issue is perhaps best encapsulated by the quote above from a letter by Dr. John Fryer, to the Editor of Lancet in the 1970's at the height of the "Death and Dying" movement started by Elizabeth Kubler-Ross in 1969 with the publication of her book, "On Death and Dying." Psychiatrists, psychologists, and other mental health professions jumped on this bandwagon to aid patients in navigating the five stages of dying that Dr. Kubler-Ross outlined in her book.

The involvement in this process became somewhat of a "cottage industry" for some mental health professionals. As with many such fads, this movement has undoubtedly helped some people who are dying, but there were some negative aspects that were lost in the enthusiasm. Most patients who are dying do not have psychiatric disorders (psychiatric symptoms or signs). The process of dying is often extremely painful, both emotionally and physically, but it is <u>normal.</u> As consultation psychiatrists, we need to ask ourselves whether we have a constructive role to play in helping patients navigate what is essentially a <u>normal</u> life process. The answer to this question is complicated, and we will discuss below some of the positive and negative aspects of psychiatric involvement in the care of the dying patient.

Our physician colleagues will occasionally ask us to evaluate and treat patients who are terminally ill and dying, and there are a number of reasons the patient's physician will seek to involve us in the care of their dying patient. The most valid reason for a referral is the presence of significant psychiatric symptoms and signs that have the potential to add a considerable symptomatic burden on a dying patient right at the time when her biological, psychological, and social reserves and resources are most challenged. Psychiatrists have an important role to play here in aggressively targeting these symptoms to decrease the overall morbidity that the patient is suffering.

There are times, however, when the motives for a referral of this type are much more complicated. Occasionally, the treating physician may feel overwhelmed by the emotional demands of the patient, or the physician may be experiencing some painful feelings of his own in caring for the dying patient. This occurs if the physician has had a long history or caring for the patient and is experiencing some grief at the prospect of losing the patient. Uncomfortable feelings are often aroused in the physician if the patient is someone he identifies with, either by age, socio-economic, or professional similarities. In order to protect himself from these feelings, the physician may refer the patient to a psychiatrist whom the physician hopes will deal with these painful issues rather than having to do it himself.

The families of dying patients often feel terribly helpless about their inability to do something substantial to help their dying family member. For the most altruistic of reasons the family of the dying patient may feel it necessary to mobilize every conceivable resource to help the patient, and this may include asking the treating physician to have a psychiatrist evaluate and help the patient deal with the emotions associated dying, even though these feelings may be quite normal under these circumstances. Although these motives are genuine and usually spring from an intense desire to do anything and everything to help their dying family member, there are some hidden concerns that must be understood by the consultation psychiatrist before proceeding further. One reason was alluded to at the beginning of this chapter. In spite of the best efforts of our professional societies and progressive elements in our society, there is still a stigma attached to psychiatric disorders and, by extension, to those of us who treat the mentally ill.

Imagine, then, how it might feel to a patient who is dying when one day a psychiatrist walks in the room, introduces herself, and says that the patient's physician/family has asked that she try to help the patient.

The patient may think, "if dying is not bad enough now they think I'm crazy, too." This is a classic example of unintentionally adding "insult"

(stigma of mental illness) to "injury" (dying). This is why it has to be carefully explained to the patient, by the physician and family, exactly why a psychiatrist is becoming involved in the treatment team.

A second concern in the process of involving a psychiatrist in the care of a dying patient is the belief shared among many physicians and lay people that psychiatrists are just more sensitive and emotionally aware than others, and it is this special expertise that they have which enables them to help the patient navigate the painful path of dying. Sadly, this belief is just not true. There are certainly those of us in the field of psychiatry who have an abundance of sensitivity and emotional awareness who can bring this valuable resource to bear with their work with their patients; however, there are also many well trained and competent psychiatrists who just do not have these characteristics. These abilities and traits (sensitivity and emotional awareness) are part of any individual's personality repertoire, but they are not necessarily learned or acquired in medical and psychiatric training.

Lastly, there is the belief among many that psychiatrists are somehow emotionally "tougher" than other physicians and bear up well under the emotional demands that dying patients place on them. To some extent this might be true, but obviously we psychiatrists are human, too, and we experience emotions as painfully as other human beings, perhaps even more so since we deal with this aspect of medicine on an everyday basis. This is what makes this type of work professionally and personally very challenging. In the words of one experienced psychiatrist who worked for many years with dying patients, "the psychiatric care of the dying patient is not for the faint of heart."

An extension of this last point is perhaps one of the most valid reasons for becoming involved in the care of a dying patient. Patients who are dying are often quite aware of how painful it is for the medical team and the family to hear them talk about and discuss their feelings about dying. They see the tears well up in the eyes of friends and family members when they begin to share with them what they are experiencing. They see their physicians scurry out of the room right after examining them thereby precluding having to listen to what the patient may want to say or ask them. For altruistic reasons patients may

want to "protect" their loved one from having to deal with these painful feelings, so they censor or filter what they say, keeping the painful stuff to themselves. This adds a terrible sense of existential loneliness to the process of dying. The psychiatrist can represent herself as someone who not only understands what the patient is going through but also as one who can "take it" and not be someone whom the patient has to protect from these feelings.

Psychological Issues Involved in Dying. It is perhaps stating the obvious to say that each individual experiences the process of dying in a unique fashion based on many obvious life factors, and this individualized experienced needs to be understood and respected. There are, however, some common themes that can be explored with patients that may be helpful. Two of these themes are Loss and Loneliness. Patients who are dying and are fully aware of what this means to them often experience a type of grief reaction to the loss of their future.

This requires a little bit of explanation. We know that we live in the present, but the present is so fleeting and evanescent that it is hard to imbue it with meaning, and we rely on our past and our future to provide meaning and structure to the present. We look forward to our future, and we spend a considerable amount of time and energy in trying to shape our future. Just reflect on the process of "looking forward" to something pleasant. It could be having dinner with a friend after work. It could be looking forward to the weekend when you have something enjoyable planned. It could be a long anticipated summer vacation or trip. It could be starting the life you have planned: starting a career, getting married, having a family, building a home, grandchildren. Looking "forward" to something in the near and long term future provides meaning and direction to what we are doing in the present. Now imagine if you are told one day that you are dying and that you have a foreshortened future, nothing to look forward to, or the realization that you will not live long enough to experience what you have for so long looked forward to. You have "lost" your future, and most patients experience this loss as a type of grief, much like the grief of experiencing the loss of someone close to you. Without the forward anchor of the future, the present becomes vague, "wobbly," and lacking in meaning. The patient grieves for the loss of his future.

Intellectually, we all know that we will die someday; we just don't know when. We know our future is "finite," but emotionally we experience the future as "infinite." The age range of the average reader of this volume is between 25-35 years. From actuarial tables we know what your life expectancy is. A healthy 25-year-old physician can expect to live another 50 years. Fifty years is a finite number, but emotionally and experientially this is an "infinite" amount of time, i.e., it is all the time one needs to construct the future life they have dreamed of and to accomplish even the most ambitious of life plans.

Consider a person in her 60's who, by the same actuarial tables, may expect to live another 15 years. This, too, is a "finite" number (rationally), but it is still experienced emotionally as almost infinite in the sense that it is still enough time to have a full "future," to continue to accomplish things, and to run through their "bucket list." Now imagine the impact on a 60-year-old that has just been told, with great authority, that all those months and years she had expected to have remaining in her "life bank" had just been wiped away by the results of a life threatening abnormality seen on a MRI scan or a blood test. The patient's future, and all the plans and dreams contained in it, has just been suddenly foreshortened, and with it the loss of what is most meaningful in life. That is why it is important to understand and appreciate how and why a dying patient is grieving for the loss of their "future."

The therapeutic challenge here is to provide some sort of short term future to give the patient a sense of meaning, structure, and direction to their life. This is not easy, but it is one of the more creative psychotherapeutic challenges we face in helping patients navigate this part of their life.

The other psychological issue often faced by dying patients is <u>loneliness</u>. This was alluded to above in the discussion of why some dying patients are referred to psychiatrists. Some patients have few people they are close to that they feel they can confide in. Others, as mentioned above, do not confide in family or loved ones for altruistic reasons: They notice how much it hurts their loved ones to hear them speak about what they are experiencing as they deal with the process of dying. The therapist who engages with the dying patient is, by her actions, saying to the patient, "I will walk with you down this path as far as you want me to." The therapist indicates by this commitment that s/he (therapist) can handle the patient's emotions (this may or may not be true, but we have to put up a good show of it). In this way, the therapist helps to diminish in some small way the terrible loneliness that certain people experience as they go through the dying process.

It is important to question the dying patient about their spiritual and religious life. If religion is an important part of their life, or was in the past, it is important to see if the patient is open to talking to a member of the clergy. Psychiatric trainees often ask, "what do I talk to a dying patient about?" "How do I treat them?" There is no set answer to this question, but it is important to realize that your job is not to <u>treat</u> them, but to respond to them and accompany them on their journey, and to help them deal with their suddenly foreshortened life.

The themes of <u>Loss</u> and <u>Loneliness</u> are but two very general themes that are often encountered, and it is a good way to start in working with a patient who is dying; however, it is important to always remember that it is the patient's agenda, not ours, that is important. Some patients will want to discuss the process of "tidying things up" in their life, have last conversations, say good bye, make amends, forgive, and ask for forgiveness. These issues are often quite complex, and the therapist can be quite helpful in assisting the patient in sorting through these issues and guiding them toward a sense of resolution. The German poet, Rainer Maria Rilke had a very descriptive phrase for this process in his *The Duino Elegies.* He called it helping the patient with a "well-crafted death," although in the context of the poem he meant a "well-crafted" end of life.

There is another issue that must be addressed here and that is "physician assisted suicide." This extremely complex issue has, over the decades, insinuated itself into the discussion of end-of-life issues. This once taboo subject has now become something that is openly debated and discussed by physicians, ethicists, lawyers, and legislators. Five states have passed legislation enabling physicians, under carefully specified conditions, to assist and enable dying patients to have the means of terminating their life. There is an important distinction between providing the patient with the means to end his/her life and the physician actually administering directly the medication to end the patient's life. In the former instance, the physician is "at one remove" from the proximate act that ends the patient's life. In the latter instance, it is the actual motor behavior of the physician that is the immediate and proximate cause that is responsible for ending the patient's life.

American society is not prepared to accept this as a legitimate role of the physician as exemplified by the Kevorkian controversy which ended in his arrest and conviction for manslaughter. Against this backdrop, however, is a long tradition in medicine of physicians using the so called "double effect" to address the suffering of the dying patient. The "double effect" was the practice of a physician administering a large dose of a medication (usually a narcotic) to target symptoms of extreme suffering (pain, air-hunger) all the while knowing full well that the dose is large enough that it may well cause respiratory depression and result in the patient's death.

The practice of using the "double effect" is a convenient conceptual conceit for the physician because s/he can consciously and publicly claim to be helping the patient by treating painful symptoms, all the while perhaps ignoring consciously and publicly the more ethically painful other half of the double effect which is causing the patient's death. One important development in the physician assisted suicide movement is that it has brought out of the closet this other half of the "double effect" and made the whole issue more ethically and medically transparent.

The reader may question why the issue of "double effect" and "physician assisted suicide" should be discussed in a chapter devoted to the care of the dying patient. There are two reasons for this. The first is that the consultation psychiatrist may be asked, depending on the law in the jurisdiction you practice in, to evaluate a patient who is a candidate for physician assisted suicide. The laws in those few states that authorize

this practice all contain caveats that the candidate for physician assisted suicide have sufficient capacity to make this decision and not be operating under the effects of a reversible and treatable psychiatric disorder. If this legislative trend continues and affects more and more states, then the consultation psychiatrist will need to expand their understanding of and practice of doing capacity (competency) determinations on patients who are candidates for physician assisted suicide.

The second reason to think about this issue is that you are likely to have patients approach you directly for help in ending their life. They may do this openly, e.g., the dying patient asking you to prescribe a lethal dose of a sedative or hypnotic that they can take to end their suffering. Or they may just ask you to prescribe a medication for a clear therapeutic reason, but there may be a strong suspicion on your part that they are doing so surreptitiously to amass a lethal amount to take when they have decided to end their life. Psychiatrists are not immune to these requests.

Psychiatrists in The Netherlands and Belgium have been involved in this issue, and psychiatrists (anecdotal evidence) in this country have been approached by patients as well. The mention of this extremely complex and ethical/legal issue in this chapter is in no way meant to suggest what you should do when you are approached with this question, but only to warn you that you probably will be asked to become involved in this issue in some way, and that you should start now in doing the hard and ethically challenging work of thinking about how you stand on this issue and how you might respond to such a request.

Chapter 12: Evaluation of the Suicidal Patient

Most psychiatrists are asked to evaluate patients for suicide in the course of their practice, but it is a frequent occurrence for consultation psychiatrists since many patients who have tried to harm themselves are first seen in hospital settings for medical stabilization, and it is during that time that CPs are asked to evaluate the patient before transfer or discharge. The receipt of a request to see such a patient is usually met by the CP with a sense of dread. This is because of the high stakes nature of this evaluation which is usually done under a great deal of time pressure. There is usually pressure from our medical/surgical colleagues to "move" the patient quickly off their service to be either transferred to another setting or to be discharged. There is little time to get collateral history about the patient. There is the pressure of evaluating a patient who may not be able to provide a good history, or who may not want to cooperate fully in giving history. And most of all, there is the pressure of the CP's worry that s/he may make the wrong "call."

All diagnostic evaluations run the risk of a Type I or Type II diagnostic error. A type I error in the evaluation of a potentially suicidal patient is a "False Positive," i.e., the conclusion that a patient is seriously suicidal and at high risk of imminent self-harm when, in fact, this is not really the case. The negative effects of a Type I error in this setting is that the patient is given treatment, either voluntarily or involuntarily, which he may not need or want. This is often associated with significant financial and emotional costs to both the patient, his family, and the health care system. Inappropriate allocation of high cost medical resources (1:1 supervision, intensive in-patient psychiatric treatment) not only drains the health care treasury of much needed money but it also imposes a painful burden on the patient and his family in terms of damage to self-esteem and trust in the psychiatric profession. These concerns are magnified exponentially when the patient ends up being involuntarily committed to in-patient psychiatric treatment as a result of a Type I error.

The Type II error is the "false negative." This error occurs when the CP concludes that the patient is <u>not</u> at high risk for imminent self-harm when, in fact, he really is. The most feared consequence of the Type II error is that the patient will soon harm or kill themselves, and the psychiatrist will be <u>blamed</u> for it. It is hard to over exaggerate how important a matter this is for psychiatrists and how much of a role it plays in how they make the diagnostic "call." This concern is quite easy to understand when you contrast and compare the possible outcomes of both types of diagnostic errors.

On the one hand (Type I error) a lot of money, lost time, and inconvenience to patient and family is wasted. On the other hand (Type II error), someone dies and the consultation psychiatrist is blamed for it. Viewed in this fashion, it's not at all hard to see why we (CPs) tend to favor living with a Type I error rather than a Type II error. There is a way, however, to partially remove yourself from the horns of this dilemma, and this will be discussed below.

First, we need to discuss what we call things. Suicidal Behavior (SB) is often confused with Self-Harm Behavior (SHB), and it is important to understand the distinction between the two. SB, very simply, is when the patient harms himself with the <u>intent </u>to die and with the <u>expectation</u> that the harm he is doing to his body will result in death. In most cases, however, when a patient intentionally harms himself, the intent, or motive, is more complex and murky. The intent may be to relieve tension (e.g.,"cutters"), or to punish themselves, or to impulsively escape some painful feelings or circumstances, or to "send a message" to someone. These distinctions are usually not appreciated by most physicians, EMTs, ER medical staff, and they get bundled up into one group with the request, "Please evaluate this <u>suicidal</u> patient." But it is the job of the CP to make these distinctions because the treatment and management of these different types of SHBs are quite different. We will discuss below some characteristics of each of these types of SHBs to help in their recognition.

There are basically <u>four</u> types of Intentional Self Harm Behaviors (ISHB). Note the qualifier, "Intentional." This is to separate this large group of behaviors from an even larger group of Self-Harm Behavior, namely, "accidental" self-harm, a type of self-harm behavior that, unfortunately, all of us have experienced. But it is intentional self-harm behavior that concerns us here, not "accidental" self-harm.

Intentional Self-Harm motivated by tension relief. This type of patient usually describes a gradual buildup of intense, undifferentiated dysphoria which reaches a peak of intensity that is relieved by superficial cutting of their skin. They often cut their wrists or arms, and it is this observation that often leads the casual medical observer to conclude that the patient wanted to slit their wrist to exsanguinate and die. Nothing could be further from the truth. In fact, they often cut themselves quite delicately with almost surgical precision to just part the skin. They often describe a state of dissociation and decreased sensation in the body part they are cutting. When they notice small amounts of blood, they experience an overwhelming and pleasurable sense of tension relief. When asked if they intended to die, they emphatically deny that is what they desired. They want relief of dysphoric tension, not death.

Intentional Self-Harm motivated by "escape." This type of self-harm behavior is extremely common. It occurs predominantly in people who have a personality trait profile characterized by immaturity, a tendency for impulsive behavior, difficulty tolerating and containing frustration and dysphoric feelings, and difficulty in postponing gratification. When people with these prominent personality traits encounter interpersonal situations that provoke intensely volatile negative emotions, they usually have great difficulty modulating those feelings and containing them in the domain of thought.

These intense feelings often "spill over" into action, and the target of the action is often the self. These people want to "escape" this emotional pain, immediately, and there is scant thought given to the consequences of their behavior. It is a perfect example of the saying, "out of the frying pan into the fire." Just getting away from the emotional "heat" in the frying pan is more important than where they land (in the fire) after leaving the frying pan. It is instructive to think of these people as being much more prone to "action" than prone to "thought." This is only one half of the issue, however. All of us have psychological "buffers" or "shock absorbers" that help us deal with the many stresses and pains of life. We call these "buffers" our repertoire of "psychological coping and defense" mechanisms. If these "buffering" mechanisms are not well developed, they are more prone to being breached when encountering a particular life stress that results in an explosion of intense emotion. An added risk factor, that is often seen in this type of self-harm behavior, is the presences of chemical substances (alcohol and other drugs) that further weakens these already shaky buffers.

The hallmarks of "escape"-motivated self-harm behavior are as follows:

- The behavior is "impulsive," meaning there is a short (seconds or a few minutes) period of time between the buildup of intense emotion and its expression in action.
- There is little, if any, thought about the reasons for, or consequences of the behavior. The self-harm act usually occurs in the immediate context of a stressful life experience that is associated with high levels of intensely painful and volatile emotion.
- An intoxicant is often present that further weakens the ability to tolerate painful feelings, and contain these feelings in thought as opposed to behavior.
- The self-harm act is produced without regard for the probability of "rescue" from the harmful consequence of the act.
- After the self-harm act, when the intensity of the painful feelings has subsided and the effects of an intoxicant (if present) have worn off, the patient may express regret or remorse about the act, and may even express shame and embarrassment at what he has done.

The important thing about this type (escape) of self-harm is that the patient does not harm themselves with the intent to die. Occasionally, at the time of the behavior, they may have a dim awareness that their behavior might result in serious self-harm or even death, but little if any thought is focused on that eventuality at the time of the crisis. These patients often state that if that death happens, it happens, but that is not the primary intent or motivation of the behavior. They just want to "escape" the intolerable feelings.

Intentional Self-Harm as a Form of Communication. We communicate in all sorts of ways, verbally and non-verbally. The lexicon of non-verbal communication is varied but concrete, and it does not lend itself to nuanced meanings; however, what it lacks in nuance it makes up with dramatic impact. There is a group of people who harm themselves as a form of communication to others, usually someone important to the patient. Two "messages" are communicated in this way: 1. "Help Me"; love me; take care of me; feel sorry for me; don't blame me; take me back, and, 2. Anger: Do you see what "you" made me do?; I'm furious with you, and I'll just show you…I'll hurt myself, then you'll feel bad and guilty. Or, both of these complex motivations may be bundled together in one type of self-harm "message."

The hallmarks that identify this type of ISHB are the following:

- The SH behavior is usually preceded by an interpersonal event that the patient perceives as a rejection or as a significant threat to the patient.
- There is usually an audience that is intended to receive the message. The SHB may be done directly in front of the audience, or it may be "staged" in such a way that the patient communicates the "message" conveyed by the SHB indirectly, e.g., by calling the intended "audience" and either telling that person what they have done or by acting in such a way that the other person realizes what the patient has done.
- Rescue. The SHB is staged in such a way as to insure the likelihood of discovery and rescue. There may also be elements of the "escape" motivation in this type of SHB as well. The important thing to realize with this type of SHB is that these people do not want to die. In fact, their behavior is "life oriented"; it is operant behavior that is played out on the stage of interpersonal relations that is designed to bring about a change in their interpersonal world, a change that is more to their liking. In addition, the use of intoxicating substance may play a role in this type as behavior by decreasing inhibitions.

ISHB as a suicidal act. Of all the patients who have suffered an act of intentional self-harm, it is the patient who has harmed himself with the intent to die whom we most need to identify. The simple and compelling reason for this is that a previous suicide attempt is a significant risk factor for a later successful suicide attempt. Aside from the patient stating directly that s/he wanted and intended to die as a result of their ISHB and may still want to die, there are some characteristics of the history of the ISHB that may constitute strong indirect evidence that the ISH act was motivated by a wish to die. These are as follows: 1. A relatively long period of time between the "idea" of committing suicide and the "act" intended to bring about that result. 2. Careful planning of how to execute the act with particular attention to attempts to "hide" the act and prevent detection and rescue. 3. Preparatory acts such as oblique references to saying "goodbye," suicide notes, giving away objects, revising or checking wills, etc.

In addition, there is the psychological context in which the idea of suicide and the act occur. Suicidal ideation and behavior usually occur in the context of a severe and chronic depression. Superimposed on this chronic, pre-disposing state may be acute or subacute anxiety, panic, or severe inner "turmoil" exacerbated by insomnia. The chronic, predisposing psychological context is characterized by two overarching psychological states: 1. Severe emotional pain (usually intense sadness) and, 2. A sense of utter hopelessness that the pain, or the circumstances causing the pain, will ever cease. The combination of intense psychic pain and hopelessness that it will ever end are crucial characteristics of the psychic "logic" that often accompanies a suicidal act.

When a CP evaluates a patient who has been hospitalized following an act of ISH, the first task is to determine what type of self-harm behavior we are dealing with (escape, tension relief, communication, or true suicide) because that obviously determines the immediate and intermediate treatment of that patient. In the discussion above that described the four major types of ISHB the impression might have been given that these are four mutually exclusive categories, each with clear shining boundaries that separate them. In reality, human psychology is not so neat and clearly categorical; it is often messy with mixed motivations causing a particular SHB. Usually, however, the careful clinician can determine which motivation appears to dominate the clinical instant at the time the SHB was committed.

At the end of the evaluation, the CP will need to make a recommendation regarding management and treatment of the patient that will occur in two time frames: 1. The time the patient continues to need in-patient medical/surgical care, and, 2. Disposition following discharge from acute medical/surgical in-patient care. The overarching therapeutic objective is to prevent and protect the patient from a repeat episode of self-harm. This is where the clinical task becomes very tricky and complicated because it implies that we can somehow predict the likelihood of another self-harm act occurring in those two time frames, and it is important to remember that we just can't make these predictions with any degree of accuracy.

There is a great deal of empirically derived evidence that supports the view that mental health professionals cannot predict with any degree of validity a future self-harm act, particularly suicide. This central fact is important since many of our management response options involve some degree of infringement of personal liberties, and the clinical challenge is to carefully calibrate the degree of infringement on personal liberty and privacy with the clear need to protect the patient from a repeat act of ISHB either while the patient is still hospitalized or immediately following discharge.

Unfortunately, far too many psychiatrists want to be "safe rather than sorry," and they are willing to accept the negative side effects of personal and privacy infringement of the patient in order to "protect" the patient from even the remotest likelihood that the patient will attempt to harm themselves again and they (the CP) will be "blamed" for it. As understandable as this may be, it is important to be truthful about our motivations in this issue: we are really "protecting" ourselves and our professional reputation in the name of "protecting" the patient when we respond in this way unless the risk of a repeat SH act is very high.

Let's look at what our treatment and management options are as we walk away from the bedside following our evaluation of a patient who has intentionally harmed themselves. We need to address two issues. The first is the "safety" concern. We need to insure that the patient is "safe" and protected from the very unlikely event of a repeat of a self-harm event while they are still in the hospital. This focuses the issue on whether there is need for a 1:1 "sitter" to be with the patient to protect them from some sort of behavior that may be harmful. It has been my experience that Residents, Fellows, and Attendings often make this decision at the "brain stem" level (reflexive) rather than the cortical (reflective) level of response. The decision to have a 1:1 sitter stay with the patient is usually made without thinking about exactly <u>what</u> they want the 1:1 sitter to accomplish and without asking themselves whether the sitter can actually accomplish the intended objective. If pressed on this question, the CP might say, "the sitter will stop the patient from harming themselves." The CP psychiatrist first needs to decide whether the patient is still at a <u>high risk</u> (note I did not say make a "prediction," since that is impossible to do) of repeat SHB in the next 24-48 hours, or as long as s/he remains in the hospital.

The next question is whether the patient is actually physically capable of harming himself in the hospital even if s/he is judged to be at continuing high risk of a repeat SHB. Or, even if the patient is able to get out of bed and ambulate, whether there is the wherewithal to harm themselves. The only time, in my 45 years of experience doing consults, that a patient has harmed themselves while in the hospital is when, on two occasions, family members smuggled medication into the patient's hospital room, the patient went in the bathroom, closed the door for privacy, and ingested an overdose of pills. In both cases, there was a sitter in the room with the patient, but the sitter did not, and in fact was not instructed to, inspect everything the family brought in for the patient, nor does a sitter routinely accompany a patient into the bathroom. The other reason often given for having a sitter in the room is with the expectation (never explicitly stated) of having the sitter physically restrain the patient if the patient becomes agitated or attempts to leave. The absurdity of this unspoken assumption is obvious when you see a young female nurse's aide who weighs 120 lbs. sitting in the room with a strong, healthy 200 lb. young man to "physically restrain" him.

There are three main problems with the 1:1 sitter scenario. The first is it is a "high resource cost" intervention. A nurse's aide is usually pulled from caring for a certain number of other patients on the floor, so there is a "cost" to these other patients who will not receive as much care as they ordinarily would. The second problem is that it is just too easy to do, and it provides everyone (nurses, medical/surgical house staff, consult residents and attendings) with an excuse for not doing the serious and difficult thinking required to determine just what kind of immediate help the patient may need. And third, there is the all too prevalent imperative to "CYA" and dish off responsibility for the patient's safety to the sitter. This enables the CP to walk off the floor feeling secure that it is now someone else's (the sitter's) responsibility to guarantee the patient's safety.

After dealing with the "safety" question, the second issue the CP needs to address is how to target the high acuity <u>risk factors</u> that may have played a role in precipitating the ISHB. This means targeting the risk factors of emotional "turmoil," or agitation, insomnia, and anxiety. These target symptoms respond robustly to benzodiazepines, and serious consideration needs to be given to administering these drugs if the patient's medical and neurological condition permits. If psychotic symptoms are present, then antipsychotics need to be prescribed. Consideration should be given to optimizing any pre-hospital psychotropic medications the patient may have been receiving.

Once the concerns about immediate patient safety and symptom stabilization have been identified and met, attention needs to be directed at the question of the appropriate setting of care for the patient after the patient has been medically cleared for discharge. The two options are <u>outpatient</u> or <u>inpatient</u> psychiatric care. In deciding between these two options, there are a number of issues that must be considered.

One overarching consideration in this equation is the finding (supported by solid evidence) that there is a high frequency of repeat suicide attempts in the 30-60-day period following an initial suicide attempt (Note: this applies to true suicide attempts, not all ISHB). Another overarching consideration is that, all things being equal (which they seldom are), outpatient treatment is generally better than in-patient psychiatric treatment since the patient can receive treatment in the context of their normal social and occupational routines. The main factor that leans in favor of in-patient treatment is the safety issue. The question here is whether the patient is still unstable or highly symptomatic, and are the causes of this instability something that can be meaningfully targeted during a short (3-5 day) psychiatric in-patient stay where the patient will be in a structured, supervised setting.

The other factor that leans towards in-patient admission is the use of the in-patient setting as a "platform" on which to mobilize social, family, and psychiatric out-patient resources. This "reason" is often derided and discounted by psychiatric in-patient staff as being a "social" (and therefore not legitimate) admission. There is some basis for this concern on their part since in-patient treatment is an intense, "high cost" treatment and should not be used to accomplish things that could be just as easily done in a less structured, less intense, and less costly way.

The problem with this argument is that social services on medical/ surgical hospitals are stretched very thinly, and the staff have little experience in dealing with a highly complex psychiatric insurance and treatment environment. This lack is coupled with the often intense pressure of bed utilization, turnover, and the need to clear the bed by either transfer or discharge make it highly unlikely that safe and clinically appropriate out-patient discharge arrangements can be made.

So for better or worse, transfer to inpatient psychiatry of a patient who has made a high <u>intent</u>, high <u>lethality</u> suicide attempt is often the default option here, not because it is the better option, but because it is the safer and more available option. If the decision is made to discharge the patient to outpatient treatment, great care must be made to insure <u>early</u> outpatient follow up. This is easier said than done because of long wait times for new patients to be seen by many outpatient providers and clinics. Ideally, a patient should be seen in 5-7 days following discharge, and this often takes effort and work on the part of the CP to arrange.

The period of time between discharge and being seen as an outpatient is a "gap" that, unfortunately, many patients fall into and become lost to follow up or, even worse, have another episode of self-harm. An argument can be made that the last psychiatrist to see the patient still "owns" the patient, and this ownership lasts until the patient is handed off to another psychiatrist who accepts "ownership" of the patient. For obvious reasons this is not a popular concept among most CPs who feel that they are only responsible for patients that are currently in-patients on a medical or surgical floor. This is understandable; however, there is legal precedent from medical malpractice litigation that supports the notion of "last tag" psychiatrist responsibility for these discharged patients during the interval between hospital discharge and first outpatient appointment.

A Risk Reduction Model for Suicidal Patients. I mentioned at the beginning of this chapter, and reprised as a theme running through the chapter, that the problem of organizing the management and treatment of the patient who is s/p ISHB around the need to predict whether the patient will attempt another ISHB is basically impossible. We cannot reliably predict that a particular patient will attempt another ISHB in the future. This notion of prediction of a suicidal act in the near future has infiltrated itself into the thinking of psychiatry to an outstanding extent, and because it is abundantly clear that we are unable to predict an act of ISHB with any degree of reliability, it has created an impossible burden for psychiatrists. It is a dark thought that looms in the back of the mind of every CP who is asked to see a patient hospitalized for a recent ISHB. In so many words, the thought is, " If the patient makes another ISH act while in the hospital (and under my care), I will be responsible for it, and I will suffer all the subsequent damage to my professional self-esteem and reputation; therefore, I must predict whether such an act will occur." This implicit message unfortunately influences the patient's care because our need to protect ourselves may negatively impact what may be best for the patient. I will discuss below a totally different concept of how to think about this issue. The model that

I suggest is more consistent with other aspects of medicine, is practical, and is clinically more relevant to patient care.

There are three separate but related concepts that bear on this dilemma: 1. Foreseeability, 2. Predictability, and 3. Risk.

All three bear on the likelihood of an adverse event in the near future. For instance, if we have a group of twenty patients who have recently made an ISHB, epidemiological data tell us that 1/20 patients will make another ISH act in the near future (following the incident ISH act). Unfortunately, this is not a reliable or actionable guess because we do not know which one of those twenty patients it will be. How can we predict, among a group of twenty patients who have recently made a suicide attempt, which one of those twenty will be the one to go on to make a future suicide attempt? We can't. But we can say that it is foreseeable that one (or more) of those twenty will make another suicide attempt; we just can't predict which one it will be. We can't hospitalize all twenty of these patients just to protect or prevent the unknown one who will attempt another ISH act, although that is frequently what we end up doing. We are more willing to accept the harm to the nineteen patients who will not attempt an ISH act than to accept the consequences of missing the one who will. This then leads to the concept of risk. We can say that all twenty patients are, to a certain extent, at risk of making a future suicide attempt. We just don't know which of those twenty at risk patients will actually make a future suicide attempt. But risk is associated with "risk factors," and many risk factors are suitable targets for immediate treatment and management.

To illustrate this discussion further, let's switch our frame of reference to another type of potentially lethal and morbid medical event, that of a cardiovascular event, e.g., a CVA (stroke) or a myocardial infarction. Clinical research in this area of medicine has identified a number of potentially treatable risk factors that are associated with a future cardiovascular event. But the presence of a CV risk factor does not predict that an adverse CV event will occur in the near future. It only says that such a future event is foreseeable or or likely to happen because of the presence of certain risk factors.

If we were to ask a cardiologist or a neurologist to predict which one of their twenty patients with CV risk factors will have a serious, or fatal, MI or CVA within a near future time frame, they would honestly say that they cannot make this prediction, but they can say that the presence of significant risk factors make an adverse future CV event foreseeable, and therefore presents an opportunity to target appropriate risk factors to decrease the foreseeability that any of those twenty patients with CV risk factors will have an adverse CV event in the near future.

Many medical specialists including anesthesiologists, cardiologists and neurologists use a process of "risk stratification" to guide them through this process. I will outline below such a "risk stratification" scheme that can be used as a roadmap to guide treatment and behavioral management of the patient who has just made an ISH act. This scheme is arbitrarily divided into four "Levels of Risk." It is important to remember that some risks are more clinically significant than others, and this means we want to identify a risk factor that is actionable, i.e., the risk factor can be modified in some way to alter the causal chain of events that leads to an adverse clinical outcome. Non-modifiable risk factors, e.g., family history of a heritable condition, may be important to note, but we can't modify a person's family history.

Level 1 Risk (Demographic-Historical). Risk factors at this level are historical and demographic, and therefore are not modifiable. Examples are older age, male sex, living alone, chronically ill, history of previous suicide attempts (or other ISHBs), and recent emotionally significant psychosocial loss. The question is, "what can we do about these risks once we have discovered them?" We obviously can't change them. But we can use the presence of some or all of this data to prompt us to adopt the posture of "vigilant monitoring." Physicians in clinical practice usually have many active patients, but the good doctors "worry" about some of their patients more than than others in their practice because they have more disease risks. "Vigilant monitoring" can take many different forms, but the basic response is to see and evaluate this group of patient more frequently to determine if they develop other risk factors at a higher level.

Level 2 Risk: **(Disorder Related Risks).** This level of risk involves those active co-morbid psychiatric disorders that are known to be highly associated with suicidal acts and which function as "amplifying" factors in the causal chain that leads to suicide. This includes Major Depressive Disorder, Bipolar Disorder, Schizophrenia, Substance Abuse, Anxiety/Panic Disorder, and severe Axis 2 Personality Trait Disorders. The clinical response to the identification of any of these disorders is to aggressively maximize the pharmacologic and psycho-social treatment of these disorders in the hopes of modifying the adverse clinical effect that these disorders may play in the causal chain leading to a suicidal act. As CPs we are often hesitant to modify the treatment plan of any patient that we see in the hospital since we have so little time with the patient. We often defer that issue to the patient's treating psychiatrist. However, I urge you to be more proactive with these patients. While the patient is in your care, he is <u>your</u> patient, and you have the obligation to maximize his treatment if you see the opportunity to do so rather that deferring that decision to someone else to make at a later time. Of course, it is good practice to communicate with the outpatient psychiatrist and discuss the decision, but it should not be deferred.

Level 3 Risk: **(Loss, Pain, and Hopelessness).** This risk level contains psychological elements of significant psychosocial loss (partner, friend, job, health, status) that leads to severe psychological pain. The psychological pain can be experienced as sadness, or guilt, or shame, or anxiety, or rage, but however it is experienced it is usually quite severe and painful. If the pain persists, it may lead to the sense of hopelessness, i.e., the conclusion that the pain will never, ever go away. This is an important evolution in the process of risk, and it needs to be clearly identified. All of us human beings have experienced pain (physical and psychological) in our lifetimes, and pain can sometimes completely fill our horizon, but usually we can bear up under it because we know or sense that it will not continue on forever. We know from past experience that something can usually be done to lessen the suffering, and therefore become more tolerable. Now imagine how desperate one might become if you are suffering excruciating pain and you come to think that it will never, ever go away.

Under these circumstances, one can easily imagine becoming desperate and thinking that suicide is a "reasonable" solution. Clinical studies have shown that high scores on clinical rating instruments that measure the degree of hopelessness are very highly correlated with suicide attempts. So the "triad" of <u>Loss</u> leading to <u>Pain</u> leading to <u>Hopelessness</u> is an extremely important risk factor. The response to this level of risk is primarily psychotherapeutic. Brief, focused reality based, cognitive and supportive therapy should be used to elucidate the underlying assumptions that underlie the patient's thinking in this regard. Rarely can you change the way a person thinks about the current situation in just one or two therapeutic conversations, but you might be able to introduce enough doubt in the patient's logic that produces a glimmer of hope, and may result in the patient backing away from the intent to kill himself.

Included in this risk level is the stage of suicidal thinking, and it is important to determine how far down the path of suicidal thinking the patient has progressed. We know from talking to patients who have made high intent, high lethality suicide attempts and who have been "rescued" that there is a certain begins with <u>suicidal ideation</u> (passive or active). Ideation then progresses to <u>suicidal intent</u>. This is a crucial step because it usually means the patient is not just thinking about suicide but "intends" to do something about it. Intention leads to <u>planning</u> the suicidal behavior, and it is important to elucidate the degree of planning for the future act. Planning proceeds to <u>acts in furtherance</u> of the plan, e.g., accumulating a lethal number of pills or acquiring a firearm.

<u>Level 4 Risk:</u> (Unbearable Turmoil/Agitation). The proximate link in the causal chain that leads to the suicidal act is often an emotional state that is variously described as unbearable inner turmoil or agitation. This emotional state is often aggravated by chronic insomnia and/or acute substance use. It is of the utmost importance to monitor patients for this because not only is it the proximate link in the causal chain of suicide, but it is the link that is most easily addressed by immediate administration of sedative drugs (usually benzodiazepines) that will enable the patient to, temporarily back away from the precipice of initiating their suicidal act.

The clinical utility of doing a risk stratification employing these levels of risk is not just to determine how high the risk is of the patient initiating a suicidal act, but it also identifies a clear risk "target" to guide pharmacologic and psychotherapeutic intervention. This scheme of risk level also has management implication concerning the most suitable setting of care for the patient. A patient at Level 4 risk obviously should be hospitalized on a psychiatric in-patient unit (possibly on 1:1 monitoring) until they have dropped back to a level 3 or 2. Some patients at level 3 risk may also need to be hospitalized if the patient is unstable. On the other hand, patients at level 1 or 2 risk may be able to be safely managed on an outpatient setting.

In summary, approach the evaluation, treatment, and management of the patient who has been hospitalized following an ISH act, not with the dread of having to do the impossible, i.e., "predict" whether you think the patient will make another suicide attempt in the near future, because this is just impossible to do. Do what other physicians do in their specialties, and perform a detailed risk stratification to identify those risk factors that we know are associated with a suicide attempt but not necessarily predictive of one. Then aggressively target those risk factors to disrupt the complex causal chain that might lead to a repeat suicidal act.

Chapter 13: Psychopharmacology in the Medically Ill Patient

It is a truism of basic Pharmacology that drugs affect the body and the body affects drugs. This simple fact takes on added significance when we use drugs on patients whose bodies are significantly altered by disease processes. The psychopharmacologic agents we use in treating medically ill patients may exacerbate underlying disease processes, and the disease processes and the drugs used to treat those diseases, in turn, may have a significant effect on the pharmacology of the drugs we prescribe. When we prescribe a psychopharmacologic agent to any patient, we need to have a clear end-target in mind, and a clear understanding of what is going to happen to that drug in its travels from a pill in a patient's mouth to its "target" destination in the nervous system.

First and foremost, we need to have a reasonable assurance that the drug we give is clinically indicated and, therefore, has a reasonable chance of achieving the intended effect. In treating medically ill patients, we are on shaky ground because the scientific basis for the efficacy of any drug is determined by clinical trials on "subjects" (not patients) who have been carefully selected to produce a homogenous group. Patients who have medical illness are EXCLUDED from these trials. So how are we to know whether drug "X," which has been shown to be effective in initial clinical trials, will be equally effective in a different patient population, particularly a medically ill population? We don't know. But we generalize its effectiveness from one population to another population that may be quite dissimilar.

Second, we need to know the ultimate target or destination of the drug we prescribe. Where do we want the drug to end up? We usually answer this question quite casually by saying, "the brain." But we really need to think more clearly and with greater granularity than this. Do we mean just the brain? Or the spinal cord? Or the peripheral nervous system. And we need to know with even greater granularity where in the brain, spinal cord, or peripheral nerve the drug will work. At the neuronal level, are we aiming for the postsynaptic membrane, the transporter protein "swimming" in the synapse, the enzymes in the presynaptic membrane, the second messenger systems in the postsynaptic membrane, or the voltage gated ion channels in the axon?

Far too often we just send off the drug into the patient's body without really thinking through these issues. We just press a button on our computer to send a script, and we hope that the drug will end up somewhere in the patient's brain where it will work its "magic" and make the patient better. In this chapter, we will review what happens to a molecule of a drug we prescribe as it travels its way through the body from the mouth to its final destination in some part of the nervous system where we hope it will exert its desired effect.

Third, we need to have a detailed understanding of the side effects of the drug we are prescribing, an understanding of the specific pathophysiology of the comorbid medical condition of the patient we are treating, and a clear understanding of how the side effects of the drug might adversely interact with the patient's underlying medical condition. To illustrate this point, let's take as an example prescribing a SSRI for a patient who is medically ill and "Depressed." Remember always that patients who are acutely or chronically medically ill are usually on numerous medications that target the basic pathophysiology of their medical illness and others that are prescribed for symptom control. The last thing these patients need is yet another medication that, alone or in concert with other medications, will add to the pharmacologic "burden" of side effects and expense. So, the bar is set a little higher in this patient population when you weigh the cost-benefit to the patient. I ask that you particularly remember that the symptom of depression is quite common in patients who are medically ill. It is important to take a careful history of the symptom of depression to determine if it is a suitable target for drug therapy. As discussed more extensively in **Chapter 5**, Depression, like anemia or hypertension, is a heterogeneous disorder with different etiologies, natural history, and response to treatment. We all know this intellectually; however, in the hustle and bustle of a busy clinic we all too often just hear the word "Depression" and (at a brainstem level) our finger hits the Rx button on the computer to send off a prescription for a SSRI that we hope will decrease the patient's suffering.

There is some well-validated, empirically derived evidence (from our own Penn Psychiatry faculty, published in JAMA) that shows that SSRIs used in mild or moderate depression are no more effective than placebo. Another well-known study (the STAR-D) showed that even in a carefully selected population, antidepressants were only @ 50% effective in treating severe depression. So we do need to resist the impulsive, brain-stem reflex of hitting the Rx button on our computer whenever our patients say they are "depressed," and do a little heavy thinking about whether prescribing antidepressants to a medically ill patient is likely to help them and whether the benefit/burden ratio is favorable. If you do decide to treat, it's important that you and the patient decide on one or two "target" clinical symptoms that you can use to track the therapeutic effectiveness of the medications in a way that will help you make treatment decisions at follow-up visits.

It is way too challenging to remember all the potential or actual adverse interactions of the psychopharmacologic drugs we use and the hundreds of different medical conditions that patients may have. For this reason, it makes more sense to first understand the four major "compartments" of general pharmacology: Absorption, Distribution, Metabolism, and Elimination, and ask yourself whether the medical condition your patient has might adversely affect that aspect of the pharmacology of that particular patient. This allows you to focus your thinking more effectively. To illustrate this point further, we will briefly describe these four compartments of pharmacologic activity and provide some clinical examples.

<u>Absorption</u>: With certain infrequent exceptions (e.g., IM sedation), the medications we prescribe are taken orally and swallowed. Think how a pharmaceutical gets from the lumen of the GI tract, into the circulation, and on to the brain. Remember that there is one cell type (columnar epithelial) that lines the GI tract from lips to anus. Columnar epithelial cells are able to transfer molecules from the extracellular environment (lumen of the gut) into the epithelial cell, and from there into the systemic circulation. But the enteric environment can be quite different throughout the gut, and this difference can affect how, or if, the drug is absorbed. Substances absorbed through the wall of the stomach and small intestine are passed into the portal circulation and pass through

the liver before entering the peripheral circulation. In this "First Pass" through the liver, many drugs are metabolized and their pharmacologic activity altered before they ever reach the peripheral circulation and the brain. There are some medical conditions that affect absorption, and the clinician needs to be aware of these in prescribing pharmacologic agents.

A partial list of these conditions are briefly described below:

The "NPO" patient. Some patients with certain GI diseases (e.g., IBD, Enterocutaneous Fistulae) are required to spend periods of time at complete "bowel rest" and are unable to take any substance (solid or liquid) that may reach the upper GI tract (stomach, small intestine) which is where most drugs are absorbed. If there is a compelling need for a psychopharmacologic agent to be given during this time period, the clinician needs to be somewhat "creative" in thinking how to get the agent into the peripheral circulation. One option, of course, is to bypass the GI tract and give the medication intravenously or intramuscularly. Some psychopharmacologic agents come in parenteral formulations, e.g., some neuroleptics, some benzodiazepines, and some tricyclic antidepressants, but most of the medications we use are not formulated in a way to be given parenterally.

If a psychopharmacologic agent is to be given parenterally, we must always remember three things: 1) the drug will not be metabolized by the "first pass" process through the liver, so the active fraction of the drug will be much higher. 2) all the "dose-response" kinetics of the drug have been tested with the use of oral preparations and not parenteral preparations. 3) FDA indications and guidance for use of these drugs usually assume the drug will be given orally, not parenterally, and this requires that you carefully document in the patient's chart the reasons why you are deviating from this guidance and what you are doing to more carefully monitor side effects and therapeutic response.

Another potential solution to this problem is to remember the histology of the GI tract that was mentioned above. Remember that it is the same absorptive cell type (columnar epithelium) that lines the lumen of the gut both above (the buccal, lingual mucosae) and below (the anus and rectum) the upper GI tract.

Certain drugs (e.g., nitroglycerin, mirtazapine) are formulated in preparations that dissolve in the mouth and are directly absorbed through the buccal mucosae. It is the same with the absorptive characteristics of the columnar epithelium in the anus and rectum. Certain pharmacological agents are formulated in a suppository form that can be inserted in the lower GI tract for absorption. Hospital pharmacies can be employed to take a PO drug and prepare it in such a way that it can be enclosed in a glycerin suppository. There are obvious concerns about doing this, since we have no idea of the kinetics of absorption by this route, but if the cost-benefit analysis is heavily in favor of attempting this, then it should at least be explored. We have tried this approach in a very small number of patients without adverse consequences. You just need not to be afraid sometimes to think outside the envelope in attempting to help your patient.

Some drugs are prepared to be dissolved in the mouth and absorbed through the buccal mucosae. Some of these drugs after dissolving in the mouth are then swallowed and enter the GI tract. The advantage of this access route is that they can be swallowed with the normal amount of saliva (or just a sip of water) and therefore are usually consider safe for patients who are NPO. Those orally dissolving medications that are absorbed directly from the oral or sublingual mucosae bypass the "first-pass" circulation through the liver and are not protein bound before they enter the CNS; therefore, they will have a disproportionately stronger effect, at a particular dose, at the cellular target. The positive effect of this is that you might expect a therapeutic response at a lower dose than you would if the same drug at the same dose were absorbed through the portal circulation. On the other hand, you might have significantly more side effects as well. This is a clinical situation where you should "start low and go slow," and carefully monitor the patient for side effects.

Patients who have had Bariatric Surgery procedures. Many patients with Morbid Obesity are receiving bariatric surgery, and a subset of this increasingly large population are likely to be candidates for some type of psychopharmacologic intervention. There are different surgical procedures used in bariatric surgery, but all of them change the anatomy (and therefore the function) of the upper GI track, and this change in function may affect the degree of absorption of oral medications prescribed. There is empirical evidence that shows, for instance, that SRIs given to patients who have had various types of gastric bypass have a lower response rate associated with lower plasma levels of SRIs implying that there is decreased absorption. These findings indicate that with bariatric surgery patients, higher doses of medications may need to be used in order to insure adequate clinical response.

pH Environment of the Stomach. There is a small subset of the drugs we prescribe that are not pharmacologically active. These drugs are known as "pro-drugs." They need to be modified in some fashion to produce a pharmacologically active metabolite. Some of these pharmacologically inactive "pro-drugs" require an acid environment in the stomach to hydrolyze the "pro-drug" to produce a metabolite that is pharmacologically active. If the pH of the upper GI tract is modified, for instance, with a widely prescribed group of drugs called PPIs, patients on PPIs may have decreased acid hydrolysis of "pro-drugs" with resulting decreased levels of the pharmacologically active metabolite. Tranxene, a sedative-hypnotic, is one such "pro-drug" that requires acid hydrolysis to produce a pharmacologically active metabolite.

The three situations described above are just three examples of a number of medical conditions that can affect just one (absorption) of the four important steps (absorption, metabolism, distribution, and elimination) that most drugs go through as they travel through the body.

Distribution. After absorption, drugs are distributed throughout the body. Most drugs are bound to proteins (globulins). It is the unbound fraction that is pharmacologically active. The process of protein binding occurs in the liver, The Bound and unbound fractions are in a dynamic equilibrium with most drugs being 85-95% bound, and, therefore, not active. Any physiological perturbation that might alter the degree to which a drug is bound to protein may have significant effects of the amount of active drug that is presented to the target neuron in the brain. One major example of this is any pathophysiological process that might affect the amount of proteins available in the liver to bind to a particular drug. Protein losing states like malnutrition, protein losing enteropathies, Nephrotic Syndrome, thyroid pathology. Or old age (not a disease state) are associated with a decrease in the synthesis of plasma proteins, and this may result in an increase fraction of unbound/to bound drug possibly resulting in an increase in side effects.

Metabolism. Drugs absorbed from the small intestine into the portal circulation go directly to the liver before entering the peripheral circulation. This is referred to as the "First Pass Effect." In the liver, most drugs are extensively metabolized before being "released" into the peripheral circulation. From an evolutionary perspective, the "First Pass Effect" can be understood as an ingenious way for the liver to protect the organism from the absorption of potentially toxic substances from the GI track. In this fashion it acts as a "checkpoint" to screen all substances that might get into the peripheral circulation, and, once there, exert a harmful effect. In the liver there are two main pathways of metabolism, one complicated and the other simple. The complicated pathway is oxidation which involves multiple biochemical steps. The simpler pathway is conjugation with glucuronide. The clinical significance of these two metabolic pathways will be discussed in more detail below. The process of metabolism is controlled by multiple enzyme system collectively called the Cytochrome P-450 System.

The steps involved in metabolizing drugs catalyzed by these enzyme systems are complex, and there are a number of factors that directly affect these processes that have important clinical significance. One of these factors is a characteristic that is intrinsic to the individual. There is variation in the genetic control of the activity of these enzymes that results in the phenotypic expression of how "fast" or "slowly" these enzymes work in metabolizing drugs. This is a rapidly expanding area of scientific study known as "pharmacogenetics." The clinical significance of this variation in the rate of metabolisms is that it may account for a significant degree of the variance in the amount of pharmacologically active drug present in the peripheral circulation. For example, a patient who is a "fast" or "ultra-rapid" metabolizer might have a lower level of pharmacologically active drug in the plasma. This might result in a delayed or sub-optimal clinical response. On the other hand, a patient who is a "slow" metabolizer might have elevated levels of active drug in the plasma with a corresponding effect both on the therapeutic effect of the drug and on the incidence and severity of side effects.

A second factor to consider is an extrinsic variable that might affect metabolism in the liver with resulting variation in higher or lower blood levels of active drug in the peripheral circulation. This "extrinsic" factor is the presence other drugs that the patient may be taking. This process is known as the "drug-drug interactive effect." Simply stated, it means that if a patient is concurrently taking one or more drugs in addition to the one(s) you are prescribing, the interaction between or among all these other drugs will not only affect the rate at which your drug is metabolized but also the rate at which many of the others are metabolized. The physician needs to be acutely aware of the clinically significant drug-drug interactions because they can have potentially serious consequences. As an example, let's suppose you have a patient who is depressed for whom you wish to prescribe an antidepressant. Let us also assume that this patient has atrial fibrillation and previously suffered an embolic CVA. The patient is on warfarin with the dose adjusted to a therapeutic INR. Wouldn't you want to know whether the antidepressant drug that you wish to prescribe has an effect on the rate of metabolism of the warfarin that the patient is taking so you could take steps to protect the patient from a dangerous elevation or decrease in the level of warfarin?

These "drug-drug" interactions are far too numerous to remember, and, fortunately, there is software that can be accessed online that informs the clinician of most of these clinically significant interactions. These drug-drug interactions should always be checked before starting a patient on a new pharmacologic agent, and this is particularly important if the patient has acute or chronic medical problems and is also taking other medications that are sensitive to variations in plasma levels of those drugs, e.g., anticonvulsants, immunosuppressants, or anticoagulants.

An issue that clearly affects the liver's functional integrity is acute and chronic liver failure. There are many causes of liver failure, but, no matter what the cause, the end result is some effect on the metabolic processes in the liver and the ability of the liver to effectively metabolize and inactivate medications. This is where things get complicated and requires some thought. It was mentioned above that some drugs are metabolized by oxidation, and that oxidation is a relatively complicated process, whereas other drugs are metabolized by conjugation with glucuronide which is a relatively simple metabolic process. If a patient suffers from some pathological process that affects the hepatocytes, it is not an "all-or-nothing" situation. A "sick" hepatocyte may be impaired in its ability to metabolize drugs, but that does not mean that it is totally unable to function at all. The mitochondria in a hepatocyte are the organelles responsible for both the synthetic and catabolic function of the hepatocyte.

A patient with acute or chronic liver disease usually has an array of serological markers indicating cellular damage (AST, LDH) and some degree of functional impairment (bilirubin, ammonia), but there are more indirect markers of the hepatocyte's ability to metabolize and inactivate drugs which is usually the more narrow concern of the CP at the bedside who is trying to decide if it is safe to prescribe a psychopharmacologic agent to a patient whose liver may not be able to efficiently metabolize the drug that is being considered for the patient. There is a rough equivalency in an injured hepatocyte's ability to synthesize compounds and its ability to break down (metabolize) a compound. Clinicians usually check a patient's prothrombin-thrombin (INR) values to gauge the injured liver's ability to synthesize proteins. If the INR is abnormally high, then it means that the synthetic ability of the liver is impaired, and, therefore, it is likely that the liver's ability to catabolize compounds may also be impaired. On the other hand, if some LFTs are abnormal but the INR is normal, this finding would lead one to suspect that the liver, though injured, might still retain enough metabolic capacity to metabolize drugs. Usually, in an abundance of caution, we start the patient on a dose of medication that is 1/3 to 1/2 of the usual therapeutic dose to see how they tolerate the drug.

Occasionally, the CP may encounter a phenomenon called "pharmacologic prejudice." This refers to the belief, held on the part of some of our physician colleagues, that drugs used to treat mental disorders are somehow more "toxic" than drugs used to treat medical disorders. We may recommend that a psychopharmacologic agent be initiated and yet note some reluctance on the part of our colleague to start it. When questioned, our colleague may say that psychiatric drugs are "toxic" (or words to that effect) and that the patient's liver, kidneys, heart, etc. won't be able to tolerate it. When it's pointed out that the patient is currently on 8-10 additional medications prescribed for their medical condition, and each of these drugs also confers some potential toxicity, equal to, or exceeding that of the psychopharmacologic agent being considered, there is still reluctance to prescribe a psychiatric drug even after a challenge to the colleague to provide an evidentiary basis for their reluctance to prescribe the psychiatric drug.

This is an example, in the field of medicine, of what we often see in everyday life, and that is "prejudice" that is the result of fear and a lack of understanding. In this case, the "stigma" (fear and lack of understanding) that is attached to mental disorders in our society has extended to the field of medicine and even become attached to the drugs we use to treat patients with mental disorders. When faced with this issue, I state that the liver is an "equal opportunity metabolizer," and I further point out that the mitochondria in the hepatocyte has no way of determining if a "psychiatric" drug is more "toxic" than a "cardiac" or a "renal" drug. Rational, scientific discussions to counter "prejudice" in medical issues are no more effective than they are in non-medical discussions, but it should still be attempted.

<u>Elimination.</u> Inactive (metabolized) or bound drugs are eliminated by the kidney. A patient with kidney disease raises the concern that drugs may not be eliminated effectively and, therefore, become elevated in the plasma. Often, this is where many physicians stop thinking. Some physicians think that just because a drug is not efficiently eliminated by the kidneys and becomes elevated in the plasma that this is, ipso facto, a dangerous situation. It's important to remember that our main concern is whether the metabolite is pharmacologically *active*, not

whether the concentration of an *inactive* substance is elevated. Most psychopharmacologic agents are fully metabolized by the liver and the metabolic products are not pharmacologically active. There are, however, some exceptions. One of these is fluoxetine which is metabolized by the liver to nor-fluoxetine which is not only pharmacologically active but also has a long half-life (@5-7 days). This fact is the primary reason that fluoxetine does not need to be tapered when thinking about discontinuing it; the long half-life of the active metabolite (nor-fluoxetine) tapers itself. Another drug that is widely used is Quetiapine, and this drug also has an active metabolite (nor-quetiapine) which has nor-epinephrine reuptake blocking activity.

Chapter 14: The Agitated Patient

Hospitals are "fragile" environments, and there are certain areas in hospitals where this is even more the case (e.g., ICUs, Dialysis Units, and Radiology Suites, to name just a few). In order that hospital care progress smoothly and effectively, patients must conform their behavior to certain routines to insure the efficient operation of certain systems of care. Whenever a patient cannot, or chooses not to, conform their behavior to what is expected of them, this creates a major problem that often requires the assistance from the CP.

The basic problem here is any type of motor behavior (verbal, kicking, flailing of arms and legs, head banging, spitting, biting) that interferes with the patient's care, the care of other patients, threatens or harms staff, or damages property becomes a psychiatric emergency. We call this type of behavior, "Agitated Behavior," but that term may not fully convey the seriousness of uncontrolled behavior in a hospital environment. When asked by a colleague for help in diagnosing and managing "agitated" behavior, the first order of business is to determine which one of two broad categories the agitated behavior falls into: <u>uncontrolled</u> agitated behavior or <u>controlled</u> behavior that is actually or potentially <u>under the control</u> of the patient. Examples of uncontrolled, agitated behavior are seen in cases of Delirium or Psychosis. Examples of controlled agitated behavior are seen in patients who are immature, impulsive, or who have severe personality trait disorders.

The approaches to the management of these two types of agitated behavior are vastly different.

<u>Uncontrolled, agitated behavior (Delirium/Psychosis).</u> The approach to the management of uncontrolled, agitated behavior depends entirely on the seriousness of the behavior as measured by the likelihood of that behavior to cause immediate or imminent danger to self, others, or property. A dramatic example that illustrates this was the patient who just returned from the operating room where a ventricular assist device

had been implanted. The patient was delirious and became agitated. He was vigorously pulling on the tubes exiting from the femoral artery insertion site. Obviously, this is behavior that must be controlled within seconds or a few minutes. The immediate response is physical/mechanical, i.e., the patient's arms must be controlled and restrained mechanically.

The second response is pharmacologic. We are taught that agitation in the context of delirium is best treated with a neuroleptic, but we must remember that even if the neuroleptic is given IV, it may take 30-45 minutes to have the desired effect, and in the clinical context of the case above, this is not soon enough. While attempting to control the patient's arms and legs, by putting him in restraints and thereby protecting the surgical site, we need to think of giving the patient something that will work in <u>seconds or a few minutes,</u> not something like a neuroleptic that will take 30-45 minutes to take effect. In the case above, i.v. lorazepam was given until the patient was stuporous. This contravenes what we have been taught about not giving sedatives (benzodiazepines) to delirious patients since it may further impair their cognition; however, in this case the top priority was to prevent further damage to the femoral insertion site and the surgical site where the device is implanted in the ventricle, which, under the circumstances, is more important than the transient status of the patient's cognition. A neuroleptic should also be given to prevent recurrence of the agitation in the next hour.

There are other medications that are also available in ICU settings that could also be considered, e.g., propafol, that will work in seconds to a few minutes. In these types of emergencies where seconds or a few minutes' count, think of the following sequence: 1) Immediate control of the limbs that are creating the harm (mechanical restraint with hands, then mechanical restraints), 2) Pharmacologic options that will work in seconds to a few minutes, and, 3) preventing the recurrence of the agitation when drug#2 wears off by using a neuroleptic that will have an effect in 30-60 minutes. If the behavior in question is not severe enough to uses steps 1 and 2, and you choose to "prevent" the behavior by the use of neuroleptics, it's important to make the primary team aware of what you're trying to accomplish and, of most importance, the time frame in which you expect to see some results.

There have been numerous times when a CP has recommended that a delirious patient receive "X" mgs of a neuroleptic Q "X" hours, and when s/he returns the next day (or preferably several hours later) to do a follow up visit, the CP is met with an annoyed primary team member who tells you that "your suggestion didn't work." When you explore this issue, you find that the patient was given "X" mgs of the neuroleptic you ordered at Noon and when the behavior recurred 20 minutes later, they concluded that the medication didn't work and was not going to work, so they stopped the medication and went back to giving the delirious patient a high dose of a benzodiazepine which sedated the patient in a few minutes. There are many reasons for this reaction, but the two most common reasons are the "unit culture" and unfamiliarity (therefor distrust) with neuroleptics. The "unit culture" issue is most often encountered in Medical, Surgical, and Cardiac Intensive Care Units where serious problems emerge requiring a pharmacologic response that acts quickly within a few minutes. ICU staff have an expectation that their medications will work within 5-10 minutes, so understandably they have little patience with medications that take a longer time to work than the ones they most often use and are familiar with. Their "unit culture" is much more comfortable with a patient who is behaviorally calm, and if the price they have to pay for a quiet patient is a patient who is cognitively impaired (as a result of a sedative) then they are willing to pay that price. In these types of units, a "good" patient is a "quiet patient" even if the "quiet" patient is quite confused.

A practical problem facing the CP in these types of situations is how much of a drug, e.g., a neuroleptic, to give to target the behavior in question. In thinking through this issue, it is important to remember two maxims. One is by Lewis Carroll who stated, "if you don't know where you're going, then any road will get you there." The other maxim is by Yogi Berra who famously said, "if you don't know where you're going, you'll end up someplace else," and usually someplace you don't want to be. Applied to this clinical problem, it means you have to be very clear in your own mind "where you're going." In other words, what is your end-point with the behavior in question? Do you want the patient to be alert but not responding to internal or external stimulation with disruptive motor behavior, or do you want the patient to be lethargic, or deeply stuporous?

Almost always, the behavioral end-point you want to achieve with the patient is to decrease or eliminate the amplitude of agitated, uncontrolled motor behavior without compromising mental alertness. This is a very nuanced and difficult end-point to reach since just a little too much medication might eliminate the agitated behavior but also compromise the patient's cognition and result in a patient who is calm but unable to fully cooperate in nursing and medical procedures. Too little medication may result in residual motor agitation that still interferes with the care of the patient. If we are using a neuroleptic, e.g., haloperidol, the immediate question often asked by trainees is, "how many mgs should I give? And how often should I give it? There is no precise answer to this question. Experienced clinicians will come up with a number, but it is only an approximate number, and at this point you need to qualify the dosage recommendation with the proviso that the initial dose you choose is a "test" dose, not necessarily to "right" dose of haloperidol to reach your end-point. You have no idea whether your "test" dose will end up being exactly the right dose, or too much, or too little. This is also the reason you should resist the impulse to recommend a "standing" dose frequency, because you have no idea if your "test" dose will be the correct dose. If it's too little, then you will be recommending that they administer a standing dose that is inadequate, or if it's too high a dose, then a dose that's too high will be administered and repeated at the dosage frequency you have suggested.

I strongly recommend you suggest to the primary treatment team a "test" dose on a one-time only basis with the statement that you will return to re-evaluate the patient at the time you would expect the medication to have its maximal initial effect (in one to one and a half hours). You can then adjust the next dose, either upwards or downwards based on the patient's initial response to the "test" dose. This is also way to keep the busy CP honest by making sure s/he returns at the appropriate time to re-evaluate the patient. Faced with this complex clinical scenario, the busy and time driven CP is usually anxious to finish the consult, make the recommendations, and get off the floor as quickly as possible to get on to the next consult that is awaiting them. They do this expecting that the primary team will do the re-evaluation and necessary dosage adjustment because, after all, the patient is their patient, not ours. I think this is the wrong attitude. Yes, the patient is theirs, but the behavioral problem is ours. We own it, and we are responsible for managing it. They have "carved out" this problem and ceded it to us. When we return in an hour after our initial test dose, how do we determine the next dosage based on our cross-sectional snapshot of the patient at that time? Once again, there is no precise "cookbook" answer to this question. If you are extremely lucky and your "test" dose has achieved your end-point, the you repeat the test dose at a frequency of every 4-6 hours.

If the agitated behavior is ongoing, then you might want to increase the second dose to 2-3X the test dose. If you have "over shot" with your test dose, then you can decrease the second dose to one-half the original, test dose. I emphasize that this is an extremely rough and approximate guideline and many other variables need to be factored into the decision such as side effects, etc. The next question is whether you have to re-evaluate the patient a third time before suggesting a standing dose and frequency going forward. Excellent clinical practice would have you harken back to high school algebra where you were taught that you need a minimum of three points in order to extrapolate the trajectory of a curve. Following this rule, it would be better to see the patient a third time before suggesting a frequency; however, we just may not have the time to do this, and you may have to base your dosage and frequency suggestions based on just two data points -- the results of the first "test" dose and the results of the second "adjusted" dose. You can then see the patient the following day and make whatever dosage ad and frequency adjustments at that time. If there are no serious side effects noted, you may want to consider erring on the side of over treating rather that under treating the patient, since the risks of uncontrolled motor behavior are greater than the usual side effects on an uncomplicated, over-sedated patient. This is particularly true if the patient is in one of the "hyper-fragile" units of the hospital such as a SICU, MICU, CCU, Hemodialysis Unit, or MRI suite.

When considering the administration of a psychopharmacologic agent to an agitated patient, there are two other issues to be considered --route of administration and side effects. In general, IV Administration will achieve effective blood levels more quickly than po or im administration. In addition, po administration requires a degree of cooperation from the patient that a delirious and agitated patient may not have. If the therapeutic objective is to eliminate the agitated motor behavior as quickly as possible, then iv administration is a better way to proceed. If the clinical situation demands that the agitated behavior be eliminated as quickly as possible, i.e., in a matter of a few minutes, then iv administration of a fast-acting benzodiazepine, e.g., lorazepam, should be given. This involves an obvious "trade-off" in side effects. By giving an "intoxicant" (a benzodiazepine) to a delirious patient who already exhibits signs of "brain failure," you are willing to accept a worsening of brain function (cognitive function) in the hopes of achieving a decrease in motor activity which, at that point, is posing more of a risk to the patient.

When sedatives are given to a patient iv, great care must be taken to avoid depression of the brainstem respiratory drive centers. This is particularly the case if the patient is already being given other medications, e.g., narcotic, which are depressants of ventilatory effort, or if they have an underlying medical condition that results on carbon dioxide retention such as severe COPD or asthma. This is because benzodiazepines depress the sensitivity of pO_2 receptors on the brain stem. If the pCO_2 receptors are already depressed and you administer an agent like a benzodiazepine that depresses the pO_2 receptors, then you are running the risk of decreasing the two "engines" that drive ventilatory effort, and you run the risk of acute respiratory compromise. For this reason, if IV benzodiazepines are required, it should only be done in an intensive care setting, ER, or where anesthesia standby is available. There are other drugs that are effective in rapidly sedating an agitated patient, e.g., propofol or dexmedetomidine; however, in most hospitals these drugs can only be administered in an ICU setting by physicians who are specially qualified to use these drugs, such as intensivists and anesthesiologists.

Neuroleptics have little or no effect on respiratory or cardiac drive centers in the brain stem, so they are safe to administer iv. Depending on the size of the patient, an initial "test" or "loading" dose of 5-20 mgs of haloperidol may be given iv as a stat dose. An interesting fact about giving neuroleptics iv is that the incidence of neurological side effects (acute dystonic effects) is much lower than when a comparable dose is given po. A loading dose of neuroleptics given iv will take about an hour for a significant effect to be seen. As mentioned above, it's important to mention this time delay to the primary team so that they have a realistic time frame to determine the effectiveness of the medication.

Ideally, it would be helpful for the CP to return an hour after the initial dose is given to assess the effect on the target system and make necessary dosage adjustments going forward. If this is not possible, then it is necessary to have a member of the primary team reassess the patient in an hour and to suggest to them exactly what should be the dosage parameters for successive doses. One concern in giving neuroleptics by any route is the effect on the cardiac conduction system, particularly in the repolarization phase that might lengthen the QT interval and predispose the patient to a malignant ventricular arrhythmia such as Torsade des Pointes (TdP). TdP is an extremely rare but serious cardiac arrhythmia that has significant morbidity and mortality attached to it. Conventional clinical wisdom has established a threshold of a QTc of 450-500 msecs that should not be exceeded. It should be pointed out that neuroleptics, especially haloperidol, do not "cause" TdP. They are a "risk factor," along with a number of other medications (e.g., certain antibiotics) that are also "risk factors." Other conditions such as pre-existing cardiac conduction system disease, hypokalemia, decreased magnesium levels are also "risk factors," and these can be corrected, particularly if there is concern about a prolonged QTc.

If IV neuroleptics are urgently required to control serious motor agitation and the patient does have a QTc close to or above 500 msecs, then a careful risk/benefit analysis must be done. If the decision is made to proceed with iv neuroleptics, then it is important to get a baseline EKG, and repeat the EKG 2 hours after administering the iv neuroleptic. Assuming that all other "risk factors" (K, Mg, other medications) remain constant, then one can try to "isolate" the effect of the administered neuroleptic on the post neuroleptic QTc. If there is a 10-20% increase on the duration of the QTc on the post-neuroleptic EKG, then one might conclude that the neuroleptic is causing too much of an increased risk to continue with further doses of neuroleptic. This complex risk/ benefit analysis must be a shared decision-making process with the primary treatment team. When there is significant doubt about the advisability of proceeding with iv neuroleptics, the question is raised about alternative medications that could be given to control agitation that would not pose such a significant risk of adding to the "risk burden" predisposing the patient to developing TdP. There are two issues here --other neuroleptics that might be "safer," and a different class of drugs (other than benzodiazepines and neuroleptics) that might be used.

There is evidence that there are differences among the various neuroleptics in their tendency to prolong the QTc; however, when you look carefully at the data, these differences are of the magnitude of a few msecs, and it is hard to imagine that a difference of 5-10 msecs is clinically significant and would make the difference between developing TdP or not.

Anticonvulsants, e.g., Valproic Acid (VPA), can be used to target motor agitation, and VPA can be administered both orally and iv.; however, VPA has its own side effect profile with effects on the pancreas, liver, and marrow which must be monitored. There is some clinical experience with using Trazadone to target motor agitation in agitated patients who are unsuitable candidates for the use of neuroleptics, but Trazadone is limited to be administered orally and it sometimes takes a few days to achieve sufficient behavioral control with the use of Trazadone.

A separate but related issue concerning the treatment of agitation with neuroleptics should be mentioned briefly here in passing, and that is the use of neuroleptics to control chronic agitation in patients whose agitation occurs in the clinical context of a chronic dementia. The issue here is the finding in multiple studies of a small but statistically significant increase in cardiovascular death in populations of agitated patients who are receiving neuroleptic drugs on a chronic basis to control agitation. This extremely important but complex clinical issue is of primary importance to patients and staff of chronic care facilities.

Controlled Agitation. "Controlled" agitation implies that the behavior of concern is potentially or actually under the voluntary control of the patient. This type of behavior is usually termed "inappropriate" behavior. Inappropriate behavior may not pose an immediate risk of harm to patient or staff, but it can still adversely affect hospital routines, patient care, and adversely affect staff morale and safety. An interesting fact is that inappropriate behavior is often better tolerated in a hospital setting than the same behavior would be tolerated in a non-medical environment. This is because hospital staff are so oriented to caring for and nurturing patients that it feels somehow "non-therapeutic" to set limits on behavior and attach negative consequences to undesirable behavior because it feels "punitive." Often you can get beyond this reluctance of staff to set limits by pointing out to staff that this behavior is the expression of a "choice," and that it is not behavior that results from a "sickness." It is just "bad" behavior.

The approach to managing this type of behavior is to help the staff set firm and appropriate limits on the behavior. This involves a three-step process:

1. Clearly describing to the patient the problem behavior at issue and how that behavior is not in the patient's interest (e.g., how the behavior may alienate and distance hospital staff from the patient right at the time when the patient most needs them). In doing this, it is important NOT to get into a discussion or an argument with the patient about whether the behavior occurred, but just to state that the behavior occurred and that it must be addressed because it may adversely affect the patient's care.
2. It must be pointed out to the patient clearly and simply that the behavior is under the patient's complete control and that, in a sense,

the patient "chooses" to produce this behavior; therefore, he can choose NOT to exhibit the behavior.

3. The patient must be told that if the behavior occurs in the future that there will be consequences attached to the behavior.

As mentioned above, hospital staff are often reluctant to attach consequences to inappropriate behavior in the hospital because it "feels" as though they are being punitive towards the patient, and this runs counter to the basic reason they are working in a hospital setting, i.e., to care for and nurture patients who are ill. This attitude often results in nurses and doctors taking a much more permissive attitude towards a patient's inappropriate behavior. As the CP involved in these cases, it's important to help support staff in the more realistic framework to view this behavior. Attaching consequences to inappropriate behavior is quite challenging, and it requires some creative thinking.

First, you must try to understand what the "incentive" is that causes the patient to "choose" to exhibit this behavior in the first place. A framework to help guide your thinking about this is the **"A-B-C" (Antecedent-Behavior-Consequence)** behavioral analysis. "B" stands for the inappropriate target behavior in question. "A" stands for the antecedents of the behavior. For example, pain or discomfort may be the antecedent to the inappropriate behavior of the patient screaming out or throwing something to get attention. "C" stands for the consequences of the behavior or the environmental response to the behavior which may be reinforcing the behavior, such as getting a lot of attention from staff. Once the antecedents and consequences of the behavior are known, then you can set appropriate consequences to the behavior.

The challenge here is to attach a consequence that is proportionate to the seriousness of the behavior. The staff caring for the patient need to know that they must follow through with the consequence should the behavior reoccur which it invariably does. The next issue is who should be the person who discusses all this with the patient. The staff usually wants the CP to do this; however, most patients are aware of the difference between consultants and the primary medical/nursing team responsible for the patient's care, and it is the primary team that has the "authority" to implement whatever consequences are attached to the behavior. The best person to have this conversation with the patient is the attending physician however reluctant s/he may be to become involved in this discussion (confrontation?). The job of the CP is to help support the attending in this job and help them rehearse a "script" to guide the conversation with the patient.

The really creative part of this process is coming up with a consequence to attach to inappropriate behavior that does not compromise the care of the patient. It can sometimes be quite challenging to devise consequences to problem behavior that is both appropriate and proportionate. But this is why this type of work is so much fun!

Elimination. Inactive (metabolized) or bound drugs are eliminated by the kidney. A patient with kidney disease raises the concern that drugs may not be eliminated effectively and, therefore, become elevated in the plasma. Often, this is where many physicians stop thinking. Some physicians think that just because a drug is not efficiently eliminated by the kidneys and becomes elevated in the plasma that this is, ipso facto, a dangerous situation. It's important to remember that our main concern is whether the metabolite is pharmacologically *active*, not whether the concentration of an *inactive* substance is elevated. Most psychopharmacologic agents are fully metabolized by the liver and the metabolic products are not pharmacologically active. There are, however, some exceptions. One of these is fluoxetine which is metabolized by the liver to nor-fluoxetine which is not only pharmacologically active but also has a long half-life (@5-7 days). This fact is the primary reason that fluoxetine does not need to be tapered when thinking about discontinuing it; the long half-life of the active metabolite (nor-fluoxetine) tapers itself. Another drug that is widely used is Quetiapine, and this drug also has an active metabolite (nor-quetiapine) which has nor-epinephrine reuptake blocking activity.

One important consideration in patients with renal failure is whether they are on Lithium. Lithium is filtered by the glomerulus into the proximal tubule where, by a process of active transport, it is reabsorbed (in competition with Na) into the epithelial cells lining the proximal tubule and back into the peripheral circulation. Any pathological process that affects the filtration and reabsorption of lithium and/or sodium puts the patient at risk for becoming lithium toxic as a result of rising lithium levels. In addition, any process that affects sodium concentration and elimination will affect how much lithium is reabsorbed in the proximal tubule. Any pathological process that results in a net loss of sodium will result in more lithium being absorbed since lithium and sodium compete for the same active transport sites in the proximal tubule. Some examples of this are sodium loss from the GI tract (vomiting, diarrhea), sodium loss from the use of diuretics, excessive sweating. In addition, NSAIDS, which are widely used, can interfere with this process by affecting prostaglandin activity which is involved in the ion transport process.

Patients who are on hemodialysis are a special consideration. The issue here is the difference in permeability of an artificial dialysis membrane and the patient's native glomerular membrane. A dialysis membrane is not as efficient in filtering substances primarily due to the diameter of the pores in the artificial membrane compared to that of the glomerulus. There is a comprehensive review of which psychopharmacologic agents are differentially affected in patients on hemodialysis (see Cohen, Psychosomatics), and this gives some guidance regarding which drugs need to have dosage adjustments made if a patient is on hemodialysis.

A Clinical Comment. This comment concerns the issue of how to dose drugs no matter whether the patient is well or medically ill. Drugs are prescribed either on a straight dosage frequency or as a PRN dosage. It has been my experience that opiate analgesics and sedative/ hypnotic drugs are most often prescribed on a PRN basis, particularly to patients who are medically ill. There are various reasons for this, such as fear of causing the patient to become addicted; however, there is also the concern, mentioned above, that psychiatric medications are often enshrouded in a veil of mystery in the eyes of many of our colleagues. This often causes them to be "afraid" of these drugs and therefore they are prescribed more sparingly. When this occurs, it may deprive the patient of relief of suffering that the medication may provide. One way to think through the basics of how we prescribe medications is to remind ourselves that most of the time medications are targeted at specific symptoms.

The obvious exception to this is when the etiology of the pathological process is known and when the medication is targeted at etiology and not symptom. Symptoms are either episodic or constant. Constant symptoms are best treated with straight dosages timed at certain frequencies based (somewhat loosely) on the duration of action of a particular drug that, in turn, is related to the half-life of that drug. Symptoms or signs that are episodic are occasionally treated on a PRN basis. This is where problems occur in providing adequate relief from suffering, which is the primary duty of any physician. One overarching maxim is that you do not want to "chase" a symptom, once it has appeared; instead, you want to "prevent" it. This should prompt you to think through the underlying process that is causing the symptom. There are two variables to consider: symptom <u>frequency</u> and symptom/ sign <u>morbidity</u>. Let's take pain or significant anxiety, for example. If a patient experiences pain once a day, and it is of moderate severity and duration, then a PRN dosage is probably sufficient. However, if a patient experiences significant episodes of pain or anxiety for most of the day, then it is better to prevent the pain by giving medication on a straight order basis.

On the other hand, if the patient experiences a very low frequency but high morbidity symptom or sign, e.g., a cardiac arrhythmia or a seizure, then you certainly don't want to "chase" the symptom, after it has occurred, with a PRN dosage. Instead, you want to prevent it, even if the event or symptom occurs infrequently. Think through the real-time process of a PRN medication given to a hospitalized patient. Let's take the example of a patient with severe anxiety or panic that is occurring 2-3 times a day, and his physician has prescribed PRN lorazepam. Let' suppose the patient experiences the early signs of a panic attack at Noon. He waits until 12:30 to see if it will go away, but it doesn't.
He rings the call bell for the nurse. The nurse responds in 15 minutes (short staffed over the lunch hour), and goes back to the nurse's station to get the medication and returns at 1PM and gives the injection. The medication starts to take effect in 30 minutes. The patient has now gone

one and a half hours being symptomatic. That's roughly 35-40% of the duration of the action of the medication.

So, in cases like this it is far better to give a medication on a straight order basis unless the symptom is very low frequency and mild severity. So these simple and mundane matters require some thought, and the four clinical situations where this scenario usually plays out is when you prescribe medication to target <u>pain</u>, <u>anxiety/panic</u>, <u>insomnia</u>, and <u>agitated behavior</u>. The basic message to remember here is to avoid <u>chasing</u> a symptom or sign. Instead, you want to <u>prevent</u> it from occurring in the first place. This simple maxim is obvious if you are a neurologist who wants to prevent a seizure, not chase it after it has occurred, or a cardiologist who wants to prevent an arrhythmia, not chase it after it has occurred. The same thinking should apply equally to pain, anxiety, confusion, or agitation.

Chapter 15: Pain

The most compelling moral imperative in the practice of medicine is the duty to relieve human suffering, and somatic pain contributes more to the experience of human suffering than anything else. All physicians are trained to recognize somatic pain and to treat it; however, the centrifugal forces of modern medicine, that have caused physicians to become increasingly specialized and sub-specialized, have resulted in fewer physicians feeling competent to practice what was once a "core competency" of all physicians, viz., the understanding and treatment of pain. This is particularly true of physicians who practice in academic medical centers where there is such a high priority attached to depth of knowledge rather than breadth of knowledge.

Physicians who practice in this medical culture are very hesitant to practice outside the "silo" of their specialty. Sadly, this is the case with somatic pain, and the management of a patient's pain, particularly if it is chronic, complicated, or atypical, is often relegated to those practitioners who work in the relatively new specialty of "Symptom Management and Palliative Care." Consultation Psychiatrists (CPs) are occasionally asked to consult on patients who have atypical pain presentations or a psychiatric history of substance abuse or some other psychiatric disorder which the referring physician thinks is contributing to the patient's pain and requests for analgesia.

There is a larger socio-cultural context in which these requests must be understood. Over a decade ago, physicians were criticized, not only by their colleagues, but by various patient advocacy groups and "blue ribbon" expert panels who stated that patients' pain was being under-recognized and under-treated. One response to this highly public outcry was the establishment of pain metrics such as the "fifth" vital sign that was recorded for all patients. As is often the case with initiatives like this, there was a slow but inexorable movement of the pendulum in the opposite direction, and the major force pushing this change is the "epidemic" of physician prescribed opioid analgesics which has resulted in overdoses, death, and large numbers of patients with chronic pain that have become addicted and dependent on chronic opioid analgesia. A physician's duty to relieve suffering, particularly that suffering caused by somatic pain, is now opposed by an equally important imperative and that is to do no harm, embodied in the Latin phrase known to all medical students, *Primum Non Nocere*. This is another factor in the reasons why our colleagues involve us in the care of their patients who have pain.

Much of what will be covered in this brief chapter has been touched on in a more general fashion in the chapters on psychopharmacology and treating the agitated patient, but I want to review some of these precepts in the specific clinical context of the patient with pain.

The first and most important issue to remember in evaluating the patient with pain is the basic pharmacology of narcotic analgesics. Narcotics have multiple effects on many organ systems: they affect the perception of pain; they affect the diameter of the pupil; they affect the sensorium and level of consciousness; they affect the brain stem ventilatory drive mechanism; they affect the motility of the GI tract. The thresholds for tolerance of these various effects of narcotics vary, but it is important to remember all this when you evaluate a patient with inadequately controlled pain.

The second thing to keep in mind is that patients request narcotic analgesics for various reasons. The obvious reason, and the one that has a clear medical legitimacy, is to relieve the suffering that accompanies somatic pain, but layered onto pain relief may be a secondary motive that is psychological, viz., to alter the sensorium and level of consciousness in a way that produces a more pleasant (and less dysphoric) psychological state. Usually, adequate analgesia is achieved at doses lower than those required to produce euphoria, or a meiotic pupil, or a narcotized bowel. It is a difficult clinical determination to sort out these effects and what the patient is really asking for when he requests increasing doses of narcotics.

As a general rule (exceptions being the chronicity of analgesia use and the degree of tolerance), if you see a patient who continues to request more and more narcotic for pain, yet his pupils are constricted, his speech is slurred, and he is stuporous, it is probable that he has enough narcotic to adequately treat pain and he just wants more narcotic to achieve a different "end point" and that is narcotic euphoria and stupor.

The third issue, and perhaps the most important one, is to first ensure that the patient's pain is adequately treated. The ideal end-point is to completely relieve the patient's pain. If that is not feasible, the secondary end-point is to diminish the pain to the point where it is tolerable and the pain does not get in the way of the patient being able to cooperate fully in his recovery, i.e., participate in nursing procedures, diagnostic and therapeutic procedures, and PT/OT. Therefore, the first task is to get the patient to understand and agree on the common therapeutic endpoint. Once the common therapeutic end-point is established and agreed on, the CP needs to understand the pathological basis for the patient's complaint.

For example, pain caused by a surgical incision that is healing normally will produce a different subjective pain "profile" than a large inflammatory mass in the patient's abdominal viscera, or pain caused by a large ischemic volume of lung tissue caused by a pulmonary embolus that causes excruciating pain every time the patient takes a breath.

Because of recent concerns about over-prescribing narcotics, orders for narcotics are often written on a PRN basis. As mentioned in some of the earlier chapters, this results in the process of "chasing" pain when what you want to do is "prevent" pain, not "chase" it. Preventing pain is best accomplished by writing for a straight (not a PRN) order of narcotics. One approach that is often used to "titrate" the dose of narcotic to the end point of reducing (or eliminating) pain is to begin with a preparation of an intermediate release formulation of narcotic analgesic that usually provides adequate coverage for 6-8 hours. This can then be supplemented with a PRN order as a "rescue" dose for "breakthrough" pain with an immediate release preparation.

When the patient is reevaluated the next day, you look to see how many "rescue" doses were required in the preceding 24 hours, and you increase the "standing dose" of the intermediate preparation until you reach the therapeutic end-point of adequate pain relief. Once there is stable control of pain, you can then consider switching the standing intermediate duration narcotic to an extended release preparation that will have a duration of action of 12 hours.

Patient Controlled Analgesia (PCA) is an example of the principles discussed in the above paragraphs. When this process is used correctly, it provides a straight order of an intravenous narcotic which can be supplemented by the patient with a fixed number of "PRNs" as "rescue" doses to target breakthrough pain that is not adequately controlled by the basal rate. A very important thing to always remember when a patient is being considered for PCA, or is already on a PCA, is whether that patient has the cognitive clarity to understand the overall purpose of PCA and has the motor ability to operate the mechanism. Countless times I have seen patients in obvious pain who were on a PCA but who were delirious and had no understanding of the fact that they could supplement their basal rate of analgesia to target breakthrough pain. In other circumstances, even when the patient knew how to utilize the PCA, their motor ability was compromised in some fashion so that they were unable to manually operate the mechanism.

Once you and the primary treatment team have achieved adequate analgesia for the patient, the next step is to immediately try to anticipate a discharge date and begin planning for how you will "bridge" the patient's analgesia requirements from in-patient status to a step down, lower intensity setting of care or to outpatient status. This is a very difficult process to predict because of the number of factors that play a role in the timing of a patient's discharge from inpatient status. One factor in this determination is the extreme pressure that hospital economics play in "churning" patients as quickly as possible away from high intensity settings of care to lower cost settings (SNFs, Rehab, and NHs). The pathological processes that underlie the patient's pain usually proceed at a slower pace than the more objective criteria that determine readiness for transfer or discharge of the patient. Careful coordination of these factors must be attempted so that there is not a too rapid (or abrupt) decrease or cessation of analgesia right at the time the patient is to be transferred or discharged.

Ideally, once a patient has become physiologically stable and satisfactory analgesia has been achieved, an attempt to <u>slowly</u> decrease the dosage of narcotic analgesia should begin to achieve the lowest possible dosage prior to discharge. Often, in the rush to "churn" the patient off the floor, I have seen the narcotics abruptly discontinued with the result that the patient then begins to undergo a painful narcotic withdrawal syndrome. In this context the question will arise concerning the appropriate "rate" at which to decrease the dose of narcotic to avoid symptoms of withdrawal.

There are two rates that are often employed. The first, and the most conservative, is to decrease the total 24-hour amount by 10% of the maintenance dose per day. This is a very slow taper and it may lag behind the more rapid pace of the factors that determine a patient's discharge, but it is highly unlikely that the 10% rate will result in withdrawal symptoms. More frequently, a 20% daily decrement is employed, and that may be associated with mild withdrawal symptoms, and it is important to warn the patient about this possibility so that they do not confuse these symptoms with relapse of the basic pathological process that caused their original pain. N.B.: the 10% and 20% rates are daily decrements that are based on the original maintenance 24-hour dose that was required for symptom stabilization. The decrements are NOT based on each subsequent daily decrement since that would obviously result in an asymptote that would diminish only at infinity.

Managing the patient with pain becomes a great deal more complicated if that patient has been tolerant to narcotics prior to hospitalization. Examples of this are patients who are on Methadone maintenance or Suboxone maintenance or who may be taking a narcotic antagonist, e.g., Naltrexone, as an adjunctive pharmacologic treatment for substance abuse. Each of these clinical situations requires careful thought and a clear knowledge of the pharmacology of these substances. Many physicians think that if a patient is on high doses of Methadone as part of an ambulatory maintenance program and develop an acute physical illness associated with acute onset of pain that their maintenance dose of methadone will also be sufficient to produce analgesia. This is definitely NOT the case, and it is important to remind yourself and the primary treatment team that the doses used in methadone maintenance target totally different end-points (decrease in "craving," emergence of withdrawal symptoms, blocking of the euphoric effects of iv narcotics) than the doses required for analgesia, although there may clearly be some overlap, and the issue of tolerance to high doses of methadone clearly muddies the water.

A final word to reprise a theme sounded above and in other chapters in this Handbook, and that is to not assume that the primary team of physicians and nurses caring for the patient know as much (or more) as you about treating pain. There are clearly some physicians who know a great deal about these complex clinical issues, but they are the ones least likely to ask for your help. It is those who are uncomfortable with their knowledge base and experience in treating patients with pain who are most likely to ask for your help. I emphasize this because many times I have heard psychiatry trainees and even attending psychiatrists defer on this subject, saying, "well, they (the primary team) are the medical experts in pain control with analgesics. They know more about this than we do. After all, we're just 'psychiatrists'." Most often this is just not the case, and management of pain with analgesics is, and should be, clearly within the core competence of the medically trained psychiatrist, especially a Consultation Psychiatrist.

Chapter 16: The ICU Patient

The experience of being a patient in an Intensive Care Unit is extremely distressing, and this must be kept uppermost in the mind of the CP when evaluating a patient there. There are many reasons why this experience is so very stressful to patients, but three primary factors that contribute to this are:

- All patients in ICU settings are <u>extremely sick</u>. This is the reason that any patient is in an ICU setting in the first place. By definition, an ICU patient is sicker than any other hospitalized patient by the very fact that the patient needs an ICU setting.
- Patients in the ICU are attached to <u>lines, monitors,</u> and <u>tubes,</u> so their freedom to move about is severely curtailed.
- Most often ICU patients are <u>intubated</u>, attached to mechanical ventilation, and cannot speak. Most patients in an ICU are in pain, are terribly frightened, and may or may not be confused. They may or may not be able to speak, and many feel completely helpless.

Because of these factors, ICU staff often refer to the <u>"ICU triad"</u> of symptoms: <u>pain</u>, <u>confusion</u> (delirium), and <u>agitation (anxiety)</u> that characterize the experience of being a patient in an ICU setting. Included in agitation is severe anxiety/panic. Most, but not all, "veterans" of an ICU experience will experience some or all of the symptoms that comprise this "triad." There is little wonder then that there is a growing literature that focuses on the psychological trauma that many of these patients experience that persists long afterwards in the expression of post traumatic psychological symptoms. In a significant number of cases, deficits in neurocognitive function can be demonstrated as far out as 12 months following an ICU stay (NEJM Oct. 3, 2013). The cluster of psychological and physical problems persisting after an ICU stay is referred to as the Post-Intensive Care Syndrome (PICS).

Many patients in an ICU cannot speak, either because they are intubated, heavily sedated, or both. These conditions make the assessment of the ICU patient quite challenging. Certain people are very good at lip reading and can conduct an interview by reading the patient's lips as they respond to questions. Another approach to take is by non-verbal communication, in which the interviewer asks yes-no questions with the patient answering with either head nods or hand squeezes. Before beginning an interview in this way, you must be certain the patient understands what is required by explaining to the patient how to communicate a yes or a no, and then it is necessary to give the patient a "test" to be sure they understand. For instance, if the patient is told to squeeze your hand once to indicate a "no" and twice to indicate a "yes," then ask them to indicate a "yes" and a "no" to see if they have it right. For psychiatrists who are trained to ask open-ended questions that may have complex answers it can be quite challenging to disciplining yourself to ask very focused and closed-ended questions, but you can usually get enough information to understand what is wrong and how you can address it.

Most ICU staff are extremely adept at targeting the symptoms in this "triad" with the appropriate medications: narcotics for pain, sedatives and muscle relaxants for agitation (particularly for the intubated patient), and various classes of CNS active agents to target confusion (delirium). Some of these agents used to target one of the symptom domains (e.g., narcotics for pain) may have unintended side effects by worsening one or more of the other symptoms in the triad, e.g., confusion. This may produce a "Rubik's Cube" type dilemma where you prescribe an increased dose of a narcotic to relieve the patient's pain only to find that you have worsened the patient's confusion. Many of these issues of treating pain, agitation, confusion, and anxiety have been discussed in earlier chapters, but what makes this so challenging for the CP is having to target all these symptoms in the same patient right at the time, in the course of their illness, when they are most fragile and vulnerable as a result of the serious, life-threatening illness that has gotten them to the ICU. An excellent discussion of these issues can be found in a recent review by Reade and Finfer (Read MC and Finfer S

Sedation and Delirium in the Intensive Care Unit N Engl J Med 2014; 370:444-454).

A specific problem for which you may be consulted is the "failure to wean" problem. This occurs when a patient's respiratory parameters have normalized to the point where they can be "weaned" from mechanical ventilation. It's one of the most difficult problems to treat in the practice of consultation psychiatry for a number of reasons. First, the patient is extremely ill, otherwise he would not need ventilator support in the first place. Second, since the patient is intubated, he cannot speak to you. Most patients who are intubated are sedated, so it is often difficult to communicate with them by non-verbal means or by writing. Third, we don't really know what causes this difficulty (failure to wean) and what the underlying mechanisms are. So, we are really working in the dark when we attempt to help the patient and the ICU team managing the patient.

If the "ventilator dependence" (VD) cannot be effectively treated, it means that the patient remains intubated for longer than he really needs to be based on normalizing respiratory physiological parameters. In addition, since being "weaned" from a ventilator is a requirement for "graduating" from intensive care management and progressing on to a setting of lower intensity of care, the ventilator dependent patient is, in effect, taking up an extremely expensive and much needed resource, i.e., an ICU bed, when he really doesn't need it based on normalizing physiological respiratory parameters.

The clinical problem presents in the following fashion. The VD patient has usually been intubated and on mechanical ventilation for a week or more. As the respiratory physiological parameters (pO_2, pCO_2, and the Pulse Ox) begin to improve and normalize, the ICU staff begin a weaning protocol which involves disconnecting the patient from the ventilator, for brief periods of time, to give the patient a chance to breath on his own without the assistance of the ventilator. During this process, the respiratory parameters are closely watched, and when the pO_2 begins to drop, the patient is placed back on the ventilator. This process is repeated several times a day with, one hopes, an increasing duration of time off the ventilator. This is continued until the patient can breathe without any ventilator support. The problem arises when the patient is removed from the ventilator but quickly begins to experience "air hunger" or the psychological response of suffocation when the objective parameters of the patient's blood gases and oxygen saturation are normal.

There is a physiological disconnect between the patient's subjective, psychological experience, i.e., that of "suffocation," and physiological parameters indicating that the patient is receiving a normal amount of oxygen. The brain "misreads" a normal physiological signal as an abnormal signal indicating that the patient is suffocating and is experiencing dangerously low levels of oxygen when that is not the case. The patient begins to breathe rapidly and progresses to hyperventilation which would be a normal motor response to low oxygen levels, but in this case the oxygen levels are normal. This is associated with significant agitation and psychological distress, and it usually results in the patient pleading, while gasping for breath, to be placed back on mechanical ventilation because they feel as though they are suffocating. In very debilitated patients, the effort involved in hyperventilating causes the respiratory muscles to become fatigued, resulting in hypoventilation which then results in deteriorating respiratory parameters. When the patient is placed back on the ventilator, the subjective experience of extreme air hunger is relieved, and the patient becomes comfortable. After one or more trials that have resulted in this scenario, the patient begins to experience "anticipatory anxiety" before the next attempt to wean is carried out. This clinical scenario clearly thwarts the primary objective of successfully weaning the patient off the ventilator.

What we think happens in this situation (although we really don't know) is that, for some reason, the "set point" for triggering the subjective psychological response of severe air hunger becomes re-set at a chemical level which is normal. In short, the brain misreads a normal physiological signal as being abnormal. There are other examples of the brain misreading a "normal" physiological state as being "abnormal," thus triggering a complex psychological-behavioral response intended to correct for the mis-perceived abnormal physiological state. Some examples that are consistent with this "model" are patients who have significant eating disorders (feeling "starved" in situations where there are no physiological parameters of starvation). Patients with panic attacks and patients with PTSD have disproportionate autonomic and psychological responses to normal situations and environments. However, it is important to remember that this way of understanding these responses, as described above, is based on an explanatory model that has not been empirically tested. The utility of this explanatory model is that it does provide a framework in which to construct a therapeutic intervention, as described below.

In attempting to manage the complex problem of the ventilator dependent patient, you need to be aware that there are two potential clinical scenarios -- 1) the patient who is alert, responsive, and has a trach, and, 2) the patient who is partially sedated and on an endotracheal intubation. Rarely are we as CPs asked to help with patients in the second scenario because it is unlikely that their respiratory parameters have improved to the point that they can be extubated for a trial off the ventilator. In dealing with the first clinical scenario, viz., the alert and responsive patient, the first step in treating this problem is to educate the patient about what is happening. You need to explain that there is a "disconnect" from his subjective experience of extreme air hunger and normal respiratory physiology. This is often a very "hard sell" to the patient because the experience of extreme air hunger often extinguishes the knowledge that, physiologically, everything is "normal."

One way to reinforce this disconnect is to make the patient aware of his monitors, especially the pulse oximetry monitor. You can move the monitor around so the patient can see it easily from his bed. You need to point out the reading of the pulse oximeter, and you need to explain what the numbers mean. I usually tell them that any reading between 92% and 100% is "normal." When the patient is about to be removed from the ventilator, he should be instructed to carefully watch his Pulse-Ox monitor, and if he should start to experience uncomfortable air-hunger with a Pulse-Ox reading between 92-100% that he is in absolutely no danger of suffocating. You should also reassure the patient that if the Pulse-Ox should drop to worrisome levels, an alarm will sound and he will immediately be reattached to the ventilator.

This approach is basically a form of simple, direct cognitive therapy where you help the patient to understand and disconnect the subjective, psycho-physiological response of air-hunger and its "meaning," i.e., something catastrophic, or telling the patient that he is suffocating and about to die. As mentioned above, this can be a very hard sell because we know that physiology and emotion speak much more loudly than an abstract thought or cognition. For this reason, it is very helpful for the CP to be present when the ventilator wean takes place so that the patient can be "talked through" the experience. Often, anticipatory anxiety begins to occur even before the patient is removed from the ventilator, which can be managed with an anti-anxiety medication given 1-2 hours before the wean takes place. Buspirone or Trazadone should be tried first since those two drugs have no significant effect on brain-stem respiratory drive centers. If a trial of these drugs is not effective in targeting anticipatory anxiety, then low dose benzodiazepines, e.g., Lorazepam, given i.m. one hour before the scheduled wean is sometimes helpful in targeting this "anticipatory" anxiety. Remember, however, that benzodiazepines do have an effect on brainstem 0_2 drive centers, and care must be taken if the patient's CO_2 brainstem drive centers are compromised either by other medications, e.g., narcotics, or by CO_2 retaining pathophysiology, e.g., COPD.

A final caveat. This clinical situation really demands that the CP be present for at least the first attempt at weaning the patient from the ventilator after the first intervention of explaining the disconnect between the experience of air hunger and fear of suffocation and what it actually means physiologically. I mention this as a reprise on the common theme that runs through this handbook, and that is the constant time pressure CPs work under. This time pressure usually means that we CPs breeze into the ICU, evaluate the patient, and then leave a complicated set of recommendations, either written in bad handwriting or in a quick "sign out" over the phone, then we leave to go on to the next patient. We assume that the ICU house officer, or nurse, or respiratory physiologist understands clearly what we suggest, has the incentive to actually carry it out, and has the time to schedule it in the face of multiple competing demands. In my experience, this rarely gets done in a satisfactory fashion. It works so much better if you, the CP, are there to organize it. The problem, of course, is that it takes time.

ABOUT THE AUTHOR

Dr. Stinnett is Emeritus Professor of Psychiatry at the Perelman School of Medicine at the University of Pennsylvania. He was the founder of the Psychiatry Consultation Service at the Hospital of the University of Pennsylvania in 1982, and he was the Chief of that Service until his retirement in 2004. Since then he has continued to be involved in the academic and clinical activities of that Service. Dr. Stinnett also established an ambulatory clinic specializing in the treatment of patients with complex, co-morbid medical and psychiatric conditions. He is the author of numerous articles in the field of consultation psychiatry and psychosomatic medicine. He is a member of numerous honorary and professional societies, including the Academy of Consultation-Liaison Psychiatry.

Made in United States
North Haven, CT
30 June 2023

38383299R00113